HOW TO SURVIVE MEDICAL TREATMENT

Stephen Fulder, MA, PhD

HOW TO SURVIVE MEDICAL TREATMENT

An Holistic Guide to Avoiding the Risks and
Side Effects of Conventional Medicine

INDEX COMPILED
BY LYN GREENWOOD

SAFFRON WALDEN
THE C.W. DANIEL COMPANY LIMITED

First published in Great Britain in 1994
by The C.W. Daniel Company Limited
1 Church Path, Saffron Walden,
Essex, CB10 1JP, England

ISBN 0 85207 279 1

Production in association with
Book Production Consultants Plc, Cambridge
Typeset by Cambridge Photosetting Services
Printed and bound by WSOY, Finland

CONTENTS

ABOUT THE AUTHOR

Stephen Fulder's work combines writing, lecturing, consultancy and research. Trained as a medical research scientist and with an MA in Biochemistry and a Diploma in Human Biology from Oxford University, he was awarded a Doctorate in 1975 for his work in the field of genetics and gerontology at the National Institute of Medical Research in London. Since 1977 he has been researching unconventional approaches to health, particularly Chinese and Western herbal remedies. He has lectured extensively in Asia and America on specific herbs such as ginseng, garlic and the medicinal effects of spices, and has appeared many times on radio and television discussing new developments in the field of plants as medicines.

His books include: *The Book of Ginseng*, Healing Arts Press; *The Handbook of Complementary Medicine*, Oxford University Press; *Towards a New Science of Health* (with R. Lafaille), Routledge; *Ginseng*, Thorsons, Harper and Row; *Garlic: Nature's Original Remedy* (with J. Blackwood), Healing Arts Press; *Ginger: The Ultimate Home Remedy*, Souvenir Press. Currently he is a consultant to the authorities and local interests in the North of Israel, assisting in the development of a new industry growing and processing plant medicines. He is married with three daughters and lives both in Oxford and on an environmental homestead in Galilee, Israel.

Important Note

The many ideas or suggestions in this book are general. They are not prescriptions, and are not specific medical advice. They must not replace specific instructions given to you by medical or alternative medical practitioners. You should consult such experts on all medical matters.

ACKNOWLEDGEMENTS

I would like to thank Penelope Cave and Carol-Ann Bernheim for valuable research assistance, Dr Samuel Reis, Dr Alice Green, Jan Resnick and my sister Adele for reviewing the manuscript, my friends and colleagues for their information and encouragement and the many patients and therapists who have related their experiences.

I have used 'he' for doctors and 'she' for dietitians, nurses and physiotherapists as a literary convenience. I wish to apologise if this usage reinforces stereotypes of the doctor as male and paramedics as female.

Stephen Fulder

Chapter One

INTRODUCTION

Do you know how to get the best out of your medical treatment?

We all enter the medical world at some time or another, where we receive treatment and advice. The experiences we have there, and our memories and feelings about it, vary greatly from person to person, time to time. We may have excellent treatment from caring and efficient professionals who earn our respect. We may be completely cured by them and, thankfully, today we have never felt better. But much too often we may be treated by indifferent and distant staff who don't give us the information, care and attention we need at such times. We may not feel fully well, or healed, after the treatment. We may not be sure if the treatment was the answer to the problem or even necessary in the first place. We may even be among the minority who experience side effects from medical treatment, where new symptoms take the place of the old ones. These have been much in the public eye recently. We have all heard stories like these:

> 'I had steroids for years for my eczema, my skin was like paper and I felt worse and worse, but the eczema is still there.'
>
> 'The physician told me I didn't have very long so why did he give me chemotherapy which made me so terribly sick?'
>
> 'I had constant pain after surgery and the physicians said they would have to cut the nerves to stop the pain.'
>
> 'The physicians didn't tell me that blood pressure drugs would have such a drastic effect on my married life.'

1

'I've been more or less permanently depressed since my operation.'

'The pills made me so tired.'

More and more people today are concerned about their health and well-being. Indeed surveys show that more than half the population of western countries are sufficiently interested in natural health to take vitamins or to read the ingredients given on food product packaging. Yet however natural-minded you are, it is more than likely that you will find yourself on the receiving end of medical treatment. At that time your choice of natural health and well-being may clash head on with drugs, hospitals and medical machinery. Your natural way of looking after yourself rarely survives the impact. This is a great shame, and completely unnecessary. For we will show that it is *especially* when you are receiving medical treatment, possibly one of the most critical periods of your life, that you need a natural health attitude to see you through. One in three of the US population, according to recent studies, use unconventional therapies of some kind. One in five of the European population have been to an alternative practitioner, one in four shop in health shops. Do they need to abandon all that as soon as they cross the threshold of the hospital? On the contrary, health products and practices are not just for the healthy. They can have a vital role to play in coping with medical treatment, and in a successful outcome and recovery.

Susan is 35 years old and married to a country carpenter, with three small children. They eat vegetarian food, some of which they grow themselves, and use home remedies, erratically, for minor ailments. Recently she developed a large abscess under her arm, after a period overburdened with work.

'I took blood-cleansing herbs which didn't help and eventually found myself booked in for an emergency operation. The stay in hospital was a torment. I felt impotent, in a health vacuum. All my knowledge and interest in natural health faded away in the bright medical world like the stars above city lights. I didn't know whether to take drugs or not; I was tired and sick and run down but I didn't know whether it was because of or in spite of them. Where were the holistic practitioners? What could I do about the rotten food? Which herbs from my garden would help me with the antibiotics? What could I do to get out of the hospital faster?'

There is a new cry for patient participation in the process of healing. A cry by those of you who want more involvement in what is happening to you. Many patients are no longer satisfied with the old unbridgeable gap between the giver and receiver of medical care, a gap that would soon lose customers to other professionals such as solicitor or accountant if they allowed it. This cry of frustration is well illustrated by the true story of Penny Brohn, who tried to take part in her own cancer treatment but was humiliatingly spurned:

'During one of the periods when I had decided to take the high-technology route, I asked one of the physicians what I could do to help myself, to put myself in the winning half of the statistics. "Nothing" he replied. Within me roared a helpless, desperate king: "Nothing will come of nothing – speak again!" But I was speechless and this man had nothing else to add. We sat gazing wordlessly at each other across the abyss, knowing neither of us had the strength to bridge it.'

What should Penny do next? What means and strategies are available to her? What can we tell Susan to remove her stress and confusion?

The purpose of this book is to make sure you get the best out of your medical treatment; that you pass successfully through this experience and are treated well to become well. Medical treatment can be the most important thing in your life while you are in the midst of it. Yet often people make more intelligent, careful and informed decisions when buying a car than when choosing to undergo serious treatment. We want to explore what you yourself can do to get the maximum benefit for the minimum risk; how you can work with the staff and the system to get better, safer, easier, more dignified and more complete care.

New opportunities

You may ask how it is possible to challenge the authority and great technical knowledge of physicians with some ideas of your own. Isn't it the physician's job to care for me? Wouldn't I need more knowledge than the physician himself in order to check things while under his care? How can I, tired and sick and helpless, challenge these masterful, bustling and healthy professionals?

In fact, new opportunities have emerged to encourage patients. Things are changing. Doctors used to be more distant, superior and unapproachable. They expected patients to beg treatment, and dutifully swallow whatever was decided for them without a murmur. The patient was not part of his treatment – it was done to him. Although medicine is still today highly technical and confusing, patients often feel freer to take part. They are becoming more active. There is today a growing mood that a patient is a consumer who should be free to choose, to question, and to select the treatment that is in his *own* interest rather than the physician's. In the new age of patient power, physicians are learning to listen. It is now up to you to take advantage of this and ask the right questions.

There is another fortunate opportunity that can help the patient today, which didn't exist 15 years ago. That is the rise of alternative or nonconventional medicine. Now there is a range of new options and choices available to all of us, options having nothing to do with physicians and hospitals and which the medical staff often do not know anything about. You can use alternative medicine in order to look after yourself during medical treatment.

More than that, the whole system of medicine which has had a monopoly in the Western world for 150 years is now being challenged by alternatives. Natural medicine, the accumulated healing wisdom of thousands of years, has now returned. In Europe it is a $2 billion industry with numbers of practitioners increasing many times faster than numbers of physicians. In the US it is also a multi-billion dollar industry with an increasing influence on health-related legislation. Three quarters of General Practitioners in the UK refer patients to alternative medicine, and the same number want to learn one or other of the techniques themselves. In the US more than ten per cent of the population pay an annual visit to chiropractors and other non-conventional practitioners. This renewal has vital importance for us because it offers us new types of tools, and professionals, to use while under medical care. If patients suffered side effects of treatment in the past there have only been two options. To grin and bear it, or to ask the physician for a different pill, which may or may not improve the situation. However now it is possible to use safe, natural, alternative techniques to reduce side effects, anxiety and pain, and to enhance comfort and healing. These methods can be used in addition to, and usually apart from, conventional medicine.

We can therefore summarise the main strategies which we discuss in this book as follows:

Self care while under medical care

There are ways, some of which have been well-researched, to treat yourself so as to minimize the chances of being on the wrong side of the statistics. You can create the mental and physical conditions to reduce side effects and speed recovery. This may include special food in hospital, vitamins while receiving certain treatments or relaxation methods to help reduce complications during surgery.

Patient responsibility

A great deal can be accomplished by employing care and prudence, by not automatically believing everything you are told, by asking the right questions, and by becoming involved in your treatment.

Alternative medicine

It is possible to reduce medical treatment side effects dramatically by using the ancient wisdoms and modern experience of herbalism, homoeopathy, acupuncture, massage, meditative techniques and so on.

Risks versus benefits

Once upon a time a fundamental principle of all medicine was *primum non nocere* – 'above all, do no harm'. However modern medicine is a rather blunt instrument, and side effects are now seen as inevitable. The principle of *primum non nocere* has accordingly been modified. It is now called 'risk versus benefit'. It means physicians can do harm provided it is worth it.

The obvious problem is that this is a compromise which modern medicine has had to adopt because modern medical treatments are rather strong and often toxic. If you kept *primum non nocere* completely, most modern drugs would be banned.

A more nagging problem with 'risk versus benefit' is that the decision as to whether a treatment is worth it for you is usually taken by someone else. Is the physician the best person to judge whether it is worth giving you pills to reduce your blood pressure even though they might make you impotent? Does the physician even know all the options, including the non-toxic alternatives, so that he can be a proper guide?

In this situation it is important to make your own equation of risk versus benefit, and for this purpose to learn as much as possible of what these risks and benefits actually consist.

Some may feel that they would rather not know; that it is better not to know too much about what can go wrong. On the other hand, the evidence is very clear that if the risks are known, people actually do better in hospital. We will show, later, that anxieties generated by lack of information are generally far worse than anxieties created by too much information. In any event, in today's climate, patients are clamoring for more information. A recent survey of thousands of patients by the UK Consumer's Association, found that nine out of ten wanted more information on their illnesses and eight out of ten wanted more information on the drugs they were getting. A survey undertaken by the US President's Commission for the Study of Ethical Problems in Medicine found that

96 per cent of patients said they wanted to know everything about their treatment. Patients are better off going in to medical treatment with both eyes open, being more communicative, more careful, and more cautious than before. Doctors too benefit by openness. It restores patients' confidence in physicians and physicians' confidence in patients.

So what kinds of risks should we consider? First and foremost is the risk that the treatment may be unnecessary or inappropriate. This is especially true where surgeons are paid on a fee-for-service basis. In the US, if surgeons change over from being paid a fee for each operation to being paid a fixed salary, the number of operations drops by a half or more. Without, we should add, noticeable detrimental effect on the health of the population. Conservative estimates including that of a US congressional committee on the subject, suggest around one third of all operations are unnecessary. So this is the first risk to be aware of.

Another risk is the possibility of new symptoms that may arise because of, and soon after, a treatment. A prime example of this is diagnosable drug side effects, reckoned by the massive Boston Collaborative Drug Survey to affect one third of all patients. The more obvious the problem, the easier it is to deal with. For if it is clear, then both you and your physician will recognise the adverse effect and shift to another treatment. If you were to come out in red blotches an hour after taking your prescription you would soon be back to your physician asking for a change. Or, at least, if they are inevitable you will know about them and can assess if the treatment is worth it. Examples of such obvious side effects are steroids and water-logging of the tissues, chemotherapy and vomiting, anesthetics and confusion, psychiatric tranquilizers and twitches.

The delayed or subtle side effects of medical treatment are of more concern. For drug companies and even the physicians don't always notice the connection between the drug and its effects, and when they do it is normally hard to prove. Doctors usually keep on with the treatment until it takes almost a mass movement of the public to stop it. Examples include increased candida infections and allergies after antibiotics, cancer caused by diagnostic irradiation, chronic illness of later life caused by drugs or by removal of body parts, internal scars causing pain arising from surgery, or depression from a wide variety of treatments. Often when a physician says 'Side effects? They're not a problem. I find most of my patients tolerate treatments extremely well', he actually means the obvious side effects — the others are out of sight, out of mind. It is the hidden ones which have to be unearthed by aware patients and practitioners, for you don't always see the damage straight away. You may feel fine while taking antibiotics, even though they are exposing you to new yeast and fungal infections which appear later.

A third kind of side effect is a result of conventional medicine as a whole, and not your individual treatment. I include here, for example, the stress, poor food, risk of infection and noise in hospitals. You wouldn't have them if you went to a health spa or herbalist instead.

The benefit aspect of drug treatment also requires some careful thought and investigation. You will need to arrive at a fair assessment of how your health will be improved, 'health' used in a wider sense, which can be termed well-being or quality of life. Will the treatment help you to function better, to do more, to feel better or to live longer? Or will it just relieve some symptoms at the possible cost of putting others in its place? Don't forget that actual 'benefit' to you may be different from a physician's definition of benefit. Some telling research has demonstrated that there is a large discrepancy between what physician and patient regard as beneficial. They both agreed only half the time about whether or not minor surgery was successful. Mostly physicians don't take into account factors like energy, mood, sociability, sex, or performance at work: aspects of life which are as important as the signs that physicians do measure such as pains, blood tests and what your cells look like.

Clearly I cannot explain how to improve the risk/benefit ratio for every treatment, and every disease. Everyone is different and needs different treatment. However I can suggest guidelines and strategies both to improve the risk/benefit ratio in your favour and to deal in a new way with any unwanted effects or discomforts that may arise during medical treatment.

Using holistic and alternative medicine to ensure safe and successful conventional medical treatment

Firstly, two brief definitions. *Holistic* means *a way of caring*, (whether it is physicians caring for you, or you caring for yourself) which pays attention to all of you: to how you really feel, to your emotional, social, sexual, psychological and constitutional picture as well as the symptoms of disease. Holistic is an adjective, describing a broad and human-centred approach to treatment. It may or may not be used by orthodox medical practitioners and is usually, but not always, used by alternative medical practitioners.

Alternative medicine is the group of *nonconventional natural healing methods* themselves, which were left behind when modern medicine grew to dominance. 'Alternative' has some shortcomings as these methods can often be used alongside conventional medicine. I prefer to use the term 'complementary' medicine rather than alternative medicine for these practices since they can be used side by side with conventional medicine in modern society rather than as a replacement for it. However as alternative is a more familiar term, it will be used in this book. Such therapies include Oriental medicine, naturopathy, herbalism, hypnotherapy, homoeopathy, the manipulative therapies, healing, and others. They all aim to amplify and enhance the self-healing capacity of the body and mind, and return body functions that have gone astray. For example a herbalist will treat high blood pressure with herbs like balm and chamomile to relax the patient, garlic to reduce cholesterol and thin the blood, herbs such as hawthorn to open blood vessels, and others to adjust the metabolism so as to remove fats. Herbalists and naturopaths will encourage vegetarianism, whole foods, fat- sugar- and salt-free diets, more roughage, and possibly partial fasting. Alternative methods require patients to work with the therapist, looking at all aspects of their mental and physical health.

The effectiveness of alternative medicine against medical side effects lies in principles which are opposite to those of modern medicine. Instead of treating a disease aggressively while ignoring or even inhibiting the general health of the patient, alternative medicine would see the patients as a human being whose life style, symptoms, constitution and susceptibilities are treated together. It attempts to restore health to the whole person so that the symptoms, including side effects, clear up along the way. For example a patient experiences headaches and nausea from a long course of a certain drug. An acupuncturist will check the function of all the organ systems by examining their 'fingerprints' on various exterior parts of the body, the tongue, the voice, the skin and the pulses. He might see that the headaches are the result of liver damage caused by the drug and he will treat the liver by needles at liver points. But he may also see that the original disease, say a bronchial infection, is still there, so he will treat that too, either after the liver or at the same time. He may also help the kidney to remove toxins and waste, both of the drug and of the disease.

Alternative medicine and its practitioners can offer you a great deal of help on how you can use diet and self-care to treat yourself. In contrast to conventional medicine which prefers patients generally to do as little as possible so as not to 'get in the way' of the treatment, alternative medicine is partly instructive. For this reason it can provide you with remedies, dietary advice and especially psychological methods to enable you to pass through a medical experience successfully and comfortably.

In addition many of the side effects crop up in the areas which alternative medicine knows best. While conventional medicine is unsurpassed at repair of injuries, and at dealing with contagious, acute and life-threatening conditions, alternative medicine is more familiar with psychosomatic (mind-body), musculo-skeletal and chronic conditions, as well as ill-health in its earlier stages. The more subtle side effects, which conventional medicine cannot completely eliminate, such as headache, nausea, allergies, malaise, impotence, irritability, muscular aches, confusion, slow recovery, and slow damage to liver and kidney, are often signs of mind-body disturbances which alternative medicine is well equipped to deal with. It provides you, for instance, with the natural means for self-care, such as the right food and vitamins to take with you into hospital. You can obtain this information from books such as this one, or advice from a practitioner. Alternatively you may need to work with a teacher or practitioner first to learn a self-care technique. For example it can be very useful to use relaxation or visualization while receiving stressful treatments, and this should be learnt beforehand. In other situations a practitioner of alternative medicine will be required to work on problems and promote full recovery during medical treatment. For example it would be very advantageous to use natural medicine such as Chinese herbs to protect and restore immunity during chemotherapy or radiotherapy.

But should a holistic practitioner use alternative medicine alongside conventional treatments? When undergoing treatment, you will be encouraged to come off drugs and toxic treatments, and replace them with the milder techniques of alternative medicine. The practitioner will often tell you that conventional medicine treats symptoms while alternative medicine seeks for a fundamental cure. Although this is true, and in many cases it would be to your advantage to take his advice, it will often be the case that you will want to continue with your medical treatment, and you should state this clearly. For example you may be receiving medical care that is helpful and necessary, and if you have a good relationship with your medical practitioner you may be rightly unwilling to burn your bridges. Alternatively, you may have made your decision on which therapy to accept, and cannot, will not – or in some cases must not – stop your treatment whatever an alternative practitioner says. In fact, you should *not* have to burn your bridges. All good practitioners ought to respect and help you whatever path you have chosen. They should see your side effect problems as an opportunity for both kinds of medical system to work in partnership. In fact, two out of three of all the clients of alternative practitioners still go to physicians.

Some medical physicians may voice the opposite concern. Why should you seek advice from a competing and non-medically qualified 'expert', when you have put yourself in their hands? Why should patients need to arrive in their clinic or hospital with a self-defence manual such as this book under their arm? Some advice on how to address those anxieties of your medical practitioner is given later in the book. Suffice to say at this point that the medical profession is supposed to approve of self-care. If patients can take it on themselves to emerge unscathed from a stay in hospital, or to eliminate side effects from a drug treatment, it can only reduce the costs of treatment, and medical people will get the credit! In the end the best physicians will be happy to help patients help themselves, and the worst physicians will not.

This brings us to the question of practitioners. The ideal practitioner for total health care would be an experienced holistic practitioner possessing both a deep knowledge of natural therapy and complete familiarity with the best of modern medical practice. However at present such people are a rare species, and you may find yourself 'dancing at two weddings' – with the alternative practitioner describing your problems in terms of, say, yins and yangs, and your physician looking at the same you in terms of bacteria. There is no simple way to bridge these worlds – but you can get the best of both. I describe how to find the best medical physician and alternative practitioner in the next chapter, for like all professionals, they vary from the dedicated, careful and competent to the greedy and inept.

Let us summarise this chapter. We saw that today there is more interest in holistic care and alternative natural health, yet a lack of knowledge about how to cope with medical treatment if it becomes necessary. As patients we need to know how to use our new-found voices and choices.

We need to know fully the benefits and risks of any procedure. If we look into all the options it is clear that self-care and holistic medicine are not simply alternatives to more aggressive medical treatment. They can also help us to come through a medical experience more easily, more safely, and more successfully.

Chapter Two

DOCTORS, DIALOGUES, DIAGNOSIS

First call – your physician, your acupuncturist or your grandmother?

Your first contact with medicine is the initial diagnosis. Diagnosis is essential for clarifying any genuine health problem and preparing the way for the right treatment. It can also give you the information to understand the treatment options available.

However all too often it leads inexorably to unnecessary or irrelevant treatment that can do more harm than good. It can be the point at which you lose control.

Diagnosis can take away from you one of the most precious things you have: your sense of well-being, of trusting your body, of being healthy without having to worry about your health. A visit to a physician mostly turns up something wrong. The physician is trained to concentrate on illness and abnormalities, and this he will usually do. Now something has changed. You have a disease. It focuses your mind on itself. Your view of yourself has another dimension, that of an ill person. Vague feelings are now organized into an illness, which even has a name, and new symptoms appear to fit the bill. To take a simple example, your occasional sluggish bowel movement, once it is diagnosed as 'constipation', requires continuous laxatives. Now you do have real constipation and without the laxatives you'll feel it.

Therefore when you have a symptom or health problem that is not serious and urgent, stop for a moment. Is it necessary to visit your physician automatically? Maybe you can treat it yourself, maybe it will go away by itself, or maybe it can be safely treated by a chiropractor or a diet? It is interesting to consider that 750 out of every 1000 adults will have some kind of symptom or injury every month. Of these only 250 will go to a physician and only ten will be referred to hospital.

But how do you decide whether to visit your physician, your acupuncturist, or your grandmother? Or all three? Unfortunately there is no brief answer to this — it will need a book of its own. Yet it may be helpful to consider the following.

The type of health problem

Dr Franz Ingelfinger, editor of the influential 'New England Journal of Medicine', once said that: 'Eighty per cent of modern illnesses are either self-limited (that is, go away by themselves) or are not treatable by modern medicine and surgery.' Modern medicine does well at treating, for example, injuries; acute infections; serious and life-threatening diseases; tropical diseases; parasitic diseases; mechanical failures, or acute psychotic and psychiatric problems. The areas which it finds hard to cure include musculo-skeletal problems such as chronic backache, slipped discs, or arthritis; chronic pain including headaches, migraine and sciatica; chronic infections such as cystitis and bronchitis; allergies including asthma; cardiovascular problems especially hypertension and atherosclerosis; neurological diseases; sleep disorders and fatigue; anxiety or depression and stress-related or psychosomatic conditions. For all these latter conditions it may be worth considering a first call to an alternative practitioner.

Your past experience

Have you had this problem before? Has it been successfully treated by a medical or alternative medical practitioner, or only temporarily relieved?

The source of the problem

Look carefully at the problem and its possible origins and patterns. Is it something sudden, unexplained and worrying? You might want to choose your family practitioner for his diagnostic skills. Is it something that seems rooted in bad habits, stress, relationships or your environment? You may want to choose an alternative practitioner for his skills at helping you overcome the root causes of your condition.

Common knowledge

What can you learn about your problem from friends and family? What is recommended by self-help groups or books and articles? Who do people in your area go to for your kind of health problem?

You can, of course, go to both conventional and alternative medicine for a first diagnosis. Only ten years ago you would have found this problematic to say the least. If you had dared to state your intention to your physician he would have reacted rather huffily with 'either him or me.' The reaction of your young local physician today is more likely to be: 'I don't know much about it, but at least it is safe, so there is no harm in trying.' Alternative practitioners too know that most of their patients also consult physicians, and they are generally tolerant of cross-consultation. The risk of going to both camps for a diagnosis is that you may end up with some confusion and doubts because of the radically different systems employed. Is my tummy ache really a yin/yang imbalance or is it food poisoning? But as you know more about each kind of medical system the confusion lessens. In any event it may be less of a risk than swallowing one system hook line and sinker.

Which physician?

You have decided to seek a medical diagnosis and perhaps treatment. The medical practitioner to whom you go is vitally important as a conductor of your treatment from the moment you walk into his clinic or office onwards. He will decide whether and how to treat you, or whether to pass you on to a specialist for further treatment and tests, and to whom. You are dependent on him to get the right diagnosis, the right treatment and the most benefit for the minimum risk. He has more influence over your well-being than any other professional, so his suitability and competence is crucial.

Physicians used to have a stature to match this responsibility. They used to represent dignity, accomplishment and learning. They had to give advice and instruction in a pastoral manner to the community. Physicians also had to be very healthy. In early medicine before the advent of statistics, physicians measured patients' functions against their own, making their own health a reference point. Many traditional societies, particularly in the Orient, also required spiritual health in their physicians.

However many of today's physicians fall short of these qualities. They become physicians as much by parental pressure, studiousness or stamina as by aptitude and inclination. They may begin medical school with humanity, have to pretend to be superhuman and end up not being human at all.

Suicide and alcoholism are three times more frequent among physicians than the general population. One in fifteen physicians in the US is an alcoholic. They are also above average in divorcing, drug addiction and going crazy. They make mistakes. When several clinicians are given the same cases the results seem frighteningly contradictory. In one such test physicians are unable to agree half the time on whether colitis patients were getting better or worse. In the US five to fifteen per cent of physicians are regarded as incompetent, according to the Public Citizen Health Research Group. Physicians tend not to accept responsibility for mistakes. They either bury them, or escape blame for failures by calling them successes. For example, when many premature babies were blinded in America in the 1960s by being put in oxygen tents, physicians said that they had succeeded in saving them, a claim which has never been tested. It is only the frequency of physicians being sued in the US that is making them a little less tolerant of each other's errors – they don't want to pay such high insurance premiums. It has resulted in doctors in the US actually covering for each other less than in some other countries.

There are still very many physicians who surround their ignorance with an armour of superiority. For example, they don't want to tell patients about drug side effects because it admits their limitations. So they state that such honesty would be bad for the patient! It is a common trap into which all professionals can fall, but with physicians it can have lethal consequences. Beware of physicians who follow fashions such as the automatic removal of tonsils, adenoids, wombs, ovaries, appendixes, ear drums or some maligned piece of anatomy without clear proven benefit to the patient. The weary drugging of the population with the 'unholy trinity' of antibiotics, painkillers and tranquilizers is due to physicians of this kind.

So what should a good physician look like? What kind of person should you seek, to avoid unnecessary and harmful medical treatment? Here are some pointers to a good physician. He will:

■ Always answer your questions and give you as much information as you request. He may not want to overwhelm you with unasked for or frightening details but he is ready to be open if he sees you are also ready.
■ Give you the treatment options and let you join in the decision making.
■ Have a good deal of preventive natural health wisdom. For example one man I know had severe stomach ulceration and went through all sorts of treatments. Just before surgery he saw a 'good' physician who told him that he should always sit down and relax completely for half an hour after each meal for the rest of his life. The patient did this, and is now getting on for 90. He always falls asleep in his chair after meals.
■ Act as a pathfinder for you, to help steer your way to various professionals who can help you. He will be well-informed enough to include alternative practitioners in his list of specialists for referrals.
■ Have empathy with you, listen to you and *hear* you. This comes from a physician being experienced in life as well as medicine. It can come from being ill himself. As one physician wrote: 'As my multiple sclerosis became more pronounced, I couldn't hide it. I decided, with some uncertainty, to share this with my patients and the usual reaction on their part was a sigh of relief. They suddenly knew I was human.'

- Be confident and calm without signs of excessive ambition, overwork, strain or exhaustion. 'Burn-out' is surprisingly common in physicians, especially among interns in hospital. Here is a list of signs to watch for indicating physician 'burn-out': sense of failure; resentment; negativism; withdrawal; irritability; tiredness; clockwatching; being absent frequently; postponing clients; poor concentration; going-by-the-book; insomnia; giving more tranquilizers; frequently suffering from sickness, headaches, digestive problems; rigidity; family conflict; heavy use of tobacco or alcohol.
- Be well-trained, experienced and competent.
- Not assume that he can treat everything. He will be modest and open enough to know both his own limits and that of modern medicine as a whole. For example he will tell you that cortisone is not a cure, it can only alleviate symptoms for a while, and you should seek a cure elsewhere.
- Only prescribe strong drugs with the greatest reluctance.

A 'super-physician' with all these qualities may not be found in your back streets. But it gives you a standard to measure your local physician by.

Naturally, you should check out the practice too. Is it cheerful and well-managed? Are the staff positive? Is it overcrowded? Is it organized financially as a corporation or, in the UK, a budget-holding practice and if so how does this affect you and the essential services which you expect? However in my view all this is secondary. It is the qualities of the physician, the man, not his practice, that count.

Which alternative practitioner?

You do not run the risk of being harmed by toxic treatments if you use alternative medicine. Yet inadequate treatment from unqualified practitioners will cause frustration and expense and prevent you from seeking the correct treatment elsewhere. Here are some guidelines on choosing an alternative practitioner.

What is alternative medicine?

Alternative medicine consists of a group of separate systems of medicine. Each has its own method of diagnosis, concepts of health and disease, and method of treatment. The major systems are:

Acupuncture
An Oriental technique in which needles are inserted at specific points under the skin to restore the normal working of organs, and general health.

Herbalism
The use of herbs and natural remedies to prevent and treat disease.

Hypnotherapy with Psychotherapy
The use of suggestion to treat illness and self-destructive habits.

Osteopathy or Chiropractic
Parts of the body are moved, manipulated or massaged to restore mobility or help repair of damaged muscles and joints.

Naturopathy
A system based on diet, water cures and methods of inner cleansing to help the body to heal itself.

Homoeopathy
A group of symptoms is treated with minute doses of the type of remedy that will create those same symptoms in the healthy.

A therapist practicing any of these methods should have been trained for at least four years. He or she will be able to give you a full diagnosis and design a corresponding course of treatment. The therapist will be able to refer you to a physician or another therapist where appropriate. For example, if you go to a chiropractor complaining of headaches, he may help with tension in the neck, but he should refer you to others to assist in reducing stress.

There are some related skills in alternative medicine which

require less training. They are more as a back-up help to your main treatment. They include:

Reflexology
Massage of special areas in the hands or feet that help specific organs.

Massage
Pressure and touch, given in a variety of ways, to relax tissues and improve the circulation.

Healing
Psychic energy is given to promote healing and recovery.

Which is the best method?

It is not at all easy to decide which is the best method for which health problem. To some extent it does not matter, as the skills of acupuncture, herbalism, homoeopathy or naturopathy can be applied, in a different way, to almost any health problem. The right specialist is more important than the right speciality; a good herbalist is better than a bad acupuncturist, or vice versa. However it is useful to be aware of a few guidelines given below. For more information, consult the author's *Handbook of Complementary Medicine*.

Therapy	Especially useful for these problems
Acupuncture	Subtle, chronic or difficult to diagnose. Pain, headache, nervous, neurological, psychosomatic. Chronic, metabolic, addictive. Fatigue, vulnerability.
Herbalism	All problems with clearly diagnosed symptoms. Mild infections, upsets, aches. Household remedies. First aid.
Homoeopathy	Children, recurring, psychosomatic. As herbalism.

Therapy	Especially useful for these problems
Osteopathy Chiropractic	Muscles, joints, mobility, rehabilitation.
Naturopathy	Chronic infections, poor health, problems of mid- or later life. Diseases of civilisation. Combines well with other therapies.

Choosing a good alternative practitioner

A good therapist should:

- Give you a full diagnosis, building a complete picture of your physical, mental and personal state of health, and understanding your lifestyle and constitution.
- Carefully examine you physically.
- Be skilled, confident and expert, with a sound clinical judgment, a good intuition and sensitivity combined with experience.
- Be ready to refer you to other alternative therapists if it is a problem which he doesn't understand or outside his competence.
- Understand conventional medical diagnosis, drugs and treatments, and when to refer to physicians and hospitals.
- Always give you advice on your diet and lifestyle, and where necessary, psychological health.
- Be compassionate and very human.
- Not be unduly expensive, and not keep you hanging on while trying out treatments.

Today, there should be a wide choice of therapists in your area. You can find their names from the *Yellow Pages*, from friends, and by calling the professional associations and asking for the nearest therapist practicing the therapy concerned. Details of the main associations are given in Appendix 2. Others in the UK are available from the *Handbook of Complementary Medicine* or other guides.

Therapists practice either alone or in clinics and health centres.

Centres in which more than one therapist is practicing can give you the benefit of the combined use of different therapeutic approaches.

As with all professionals, choose by reputation, qualifications, experience and intuition.

Reputation

Ask friends and colleagues, or ask therapists of different specialities, or your local General Practitioner.

Qualifications

The main minimum qualifications of the major therapies are: *acupuncture* – Lic Ac., B Ac.; *herbalism* – MNIMH, ND; *homoeopathy* – several titles of the form: xxxx.Hom; *naturopathy* – ND, DO; *osteopathy* – DO; *chiropractic* – DC. On the other hand this is not a definitive guide as therapists add other letters to their names, sometimes in place of the above, indicating membership of professional organisations. You need to be sure that the therapist has been to one of the leading schools, which teach four year courses. You should be careful of therapists who have only learned from correspondence courses, no matter how fancy the diploma on the wall. If in doubt, contact or look up the professional association to which the therapist concerned belongs. Do not go to therapists who do not belong to any professional body.

In the case of the subsidiary therapies, such as reflexology, questions of qualification do not apply.

Experience

This means at least three years in practice. A full timer will obviously be more experienced than a part timer.

Intuition

Go and see the therapist and the centre. How do you feel there? Do you get on with the therapist? Does he inspire confidence? Does he meet your eyes and relate to you as a person?

Visiting your physician

The dialogue with the physician is your entry to the world of medical procedures. Since it is not exactly an entrance into a garden, rather into an unknown passageway, you should tread carefully. The gate tends to shut behind you – an Rx/prescription, a letter to the specialist, an order for tests, and hidden notes in your record can be scribbled, irreversibly, sometimes when you've hardly opened your mouth.

This consultation is not always easy and equal: you may not feel confident enough to ask the kind of questions which we discuss below.

The physician is still a figure of authority and power who holds mysterious technical knowledge. The patient usually comes submissively for help, begging some of this knowledge. The patient may be weak, exhausted, ill or anxious. The end result is that patients don't share in the making of medical decisions. The father of a colleague woke up one day blind in one eye. Physicians treated him for two years, without much success. He still doesn't know why it happened and is afraid to ask in case it upsets his physician.

Similarly, medical professionals can be so dominant that patients won't even accept that they can make mistakes like all other human beings. I have a friend, now over 90, who broke her femur 20 years ago. She was given a 'Girdlestone' operation, an out-of-date procedure which made a total mess of her hip. Then followed endless hospitalizations as they tried unsuccessfully to put in pins, take them out, repair previous mistakes and so on. This otherwise healthy lady became disabled but she would never once admit that the physicians might have erred. Even if all the evidence is presented to her she will say it is 'just one of those things' and 'the doctors were wonderful'.

You may well be thinking at this point that surely the physician needs his authority, since it is part of the natural relationship between practitioner and patient. Trust is obviously necessary otherwise no-one would let a physician near them and the whole medical system would grind to a halt. More than that, trust or belief that the physician will make you better (the 'placebo effect') is itself therapeutic. All this is quite true. However because modern medicine is so potent, such a two-edged sword, it is necessary to be cautious and to make careful choices. This is no place for blind faith. You should trust your physician, but only when you are satisfied that the trust is deserved.

Information is good medicine

It will be emphasised again and again in this book that information is the key to caring for yourself and getting the best from your medical treatment. Without it, you cannot know the risks of any procedure and what your options are. Your questions lift the veil from all those mysterious professional decisions and manipulations, and help you to be in control of what happens to you. Your dialogues help to keep a continuous check on whether your treatment is to your real and lasting benefit.

For example, I received this letter from Maureen, a 58-year-old Oxford woman.

'When I needed help for depression following deaths in the family, my physician gave me antidepressants and five Valium a day. I didn't take the Valium and managed to get off the anti-depressants after a year, but my freedom was marred by bouts of tiredness – I could curl up on a roundabout and sleep like a log – plus a great deal of trouble with my digestive system. My physician tended to give you analgesics for pains, anti-biotics for sore throats and coughs, and anti-depressants for anything else. When I asked for help as far as nutrition was concerned he said "You're the expert with that."

The physician gave me a regular antacid and said I was making too much acid. I grew more tired and he decided to send me to a specialist. Then began a series of X-rays, barium enema, blood tests, and an endoscopy (internal examination from mouth to duodenum). The only thing they could say was I had an inflamed gut throughout. "The duodenum seemed to resent the intrusion of the endoscope." I was put on a course of an antispasmodic ('Colofac' – equivalent to 'Lomotil' in the

US) to relax the intestinal muscles. I felt better, then worse, then better, then worse, and started and stopped with the pills repeatedly. Once, while waiting to see the specialist I listened to the conversations of the other patients. They were all on the same pills! And some of them had had several endoscopies! That did it. The next day I saw a homoeopathic physician. She examined me thoroughly looking at all aspects of my health and my life. For the first time I received some real guidance. For example, she told me that whenever I felt in need of a "pill" I should take a little honey in water, and a teaspoon of brandy, and go for a brisk walk of at least half a mile.'

Maureen was cured in a relatively short time and went back to see the specialist.

'I felt fine and was signed off by the specialist in two minutes. He just grimaced when I started to tell him about my homoeopathic treatment!'

Maureen was caught up in an inexorable medical process that was clearly doing her harm and not curing her. She wasn't happy with the situation – she tried to get off her drugs – but succeeded only in yo-yoing on and off them. This was because Maureen believed her physician's view that her tiredness and digestive problems were all due to some abnormal intestinal function. Even when the medicines didn't make her better she believed him. She should have questioned this logic. Indeed she might have found out that tiredness and digestive problems are a common side effect of the antidepressants, and that antacids are not a substitute for psychotherapy. This information should have been offered by the physician, but was not.

How to get the information you need

These are typical fob-offs recorded from actual conversations:

'Just leave everything to me, I'll take care of it all.'

'You've done too much reading' (to a girl who asked to see her x-rays).

'I do not think a worried sister will be the best help for him' (to a sister who asked the psychiatric clinic physician what drugs her brother was getting).

'I don't have time to give you lessons!'

'Don't concern yourself about the details. That's our job.'

'It's thrombophlebitis, you see' (to an uneducated lady).

'I don't discuss diagnostic possibilities.'

'Better take it out now and live happily ever after' (regarding a highly malignant cancer).

What do you do with such statements? They are worse than useless to you; a closed door. You should open the dialogue by a polite invitation:

'Please tell me what you mean.'

'I am quite capable of understanding you. I am an adult and I need to know.'

'I will be anxious unless I know all the facts.'

'It is my disease, it has happened to me and I must know about it and how to deal with it.'

'You won't upset me. I can take it, and I need to know in order to make the proper decisions.'

'Do you agree that we must work together to get me back on my feet? We cannot work together if I don't know what's going on.'

To put yourself in the right frame of mind, keep remembering that *you* are *his* employer.

You should know that *you have a right to be informed of the real risks* of a particular treatment and a physician can be regarded as negligent under the law if he fails to warn a patient about them.

The crucial decisions should rest with patients and only in exceptional circumstances should they be kept in the dark about the true state of their health or about the treatment proposed. So says the Department of Health in the UK. 'The patient has the right to obtain from his physician complete current information concerning his diagnosis, treatment and prognosis in terms the patient can reasonably be expected to understand...' So says the Patient's Bill of Rights of the American Hospital Association.

Therefore, if you do not get the information you need you can use your 'patient's power' to tell the physician that it is his duty to give you this information. But it may not be worth it. If the physician is evasive, dismissive, aggressive, or uncommunicative even after your requests, you should consider changing to another physician.

Hopefully you will not encounter such problems in obtaining full information. Indeed today physicians are being taught to be partners rather than distant professionals. *In contemporary culture it is appropriate for physician and patient to meet as equals, with the former rendering expert advice and the latter bearing ultimate responsibility for deciding whether or not to follow that advice.* This is written in a current clinical physicians' manual. I carried out a 'straw poll' among several local physicians and asked them how much they told patients about possible side effects of drugs they prescribed. The response of one doctor was typical. She said that she would always tell patients about side effects that would definitely happen. She would only give patients information on side effects that might happen if she felt they could manage this information. If not, she would ask the patient to come back for a check within 48 hours.

The actual questions to ask your physician will be discussed below in the appropriate sections. In general they are:

What is your diagnosis? Are there any other possibilities?

What are the treatment options?

What are the risks involved in each and the side effects?

How can I reduce any adverse effects?

How long will I have to take the medicine?
What will happen if I delay treatment or do nothing?
Why have I got this condition?
What self-care methods can you recommend, including diet or supplements?

Your dialogue should deal fully with these questions. But there is more. For you have a better chance of not receiving unnecessary treatments if your physician knows you. Talk to him. Tell him that you are a natural-minded person, you don't like to take drugs and you prefer preventive measures in health care. Let him get to know your life and your problems. He will see you as a human being, not a cipher. Treat him as a person too. Put yourself in his position. A more personal relationship breaks the pattern of production-line medicine. It will protect you, and by the way, help your physician to be a better physician.

Diagnosis – getting it right

It may seem the most natural and harmless activity – a doctor checking to identify what is wrong with you. Unfortunately it is not so free of risks as it seems. As the risks are less visible you should know what these are and how to avoid them.

Six years ago a 19-year-old girl of my acquaintance – call her Jackie – feared that she might have become pregnant. She gave a urine sample and the lab test was positive. However her doctor couldn't find any sign of pregnancy so he sent her to the hospital in case she had an ectopic pregnancy (a dangerous condition where the foetus grows outside the womb). The hospital whisked her upstairs for a laparoscopy (inspection of the abdomen through a surgically inserted tube) under general anaesthetic. Her lungs collapsed, her heart stopped, and the anaesthetists and doctors had to fight for her life. She was under anaesthetic for eleven hours, and in intensive care. Thankfully she recovered relatively quickly and went home. Two weeks later she received a letter from the hospital: sorry, this was a laboratory error, the original test was negative. Incredibly the same thing happened a month later to a friend of hers who had received a positive pregnancy test from the same lab. The hospital was just about to do a laparoscopy to check for an ectopic pregnancy when she reminded them of Jackie's case – they had already forgotten. 'Oh!' said the doctor, 'yes, we had better check the lab test, hadn't we?' Again it was an error.

This is an extreme case. But it illustrates the major risk in diagnosis – error. There has always been a possibility of your doctor making mistakes in clinical judgment. But today lab tests and instrumentation have replaced some of his senses, his judgment and his intuition. They can lead to much more misdiagnosis. The Centre for Disease Control in Georgia, US, has found that around one quarter of all laboratory test results are in error. In the UK, of 200 patients who had abnormal tests, only two thirds had the same result on retesting elsewhere – the rest were quite normal! The US Congress has investigated the situation: 'Faulty lab procedures can have devastating consequences for the unsuspecting' stated Democratic Senator Carl Levin of Michigan.

Hospitals as a whole tend to misdiagnose a great deal, through tired doctors relying on test results and instruments. A study of an average American hospital found that heart attacks were misdiagnosed in almost half of all cases. In general misdiagnosis is thought to contribute to ten per cent of all patient deaths in hospital (see page 42).

Even if a lab test was technically correct, risks arise because lab tests, and the hospitals and clinics which order them, are impersonal. Diagnosis is therefore based on the average within the general population. Something unusual may crop up and a hospital doctor will treat you as sick even if a doctor who knew you would know you are well. If tests are normal you could be dismissed as healthy even though your family doctor might know you are ill.

For example, a high white blood cell count can lead to all sorts of scary tests, although it could be normal for you because you are smoking heavily. Unusual traces on the electroencephalogram (EEG) have led to vague diagnoses of organic brain disease in healthy but unruly children, turning them into medical cases.

Fluctuations on an electrocardiogram (ECG) can start the whole coronary care colossus in motion, with its uncomfortable and even risky tests. Yet the ECG can vary because of the time of day, and is often misread. High blood pressure readings can lead to toxic medication. However it is known that blood pressure increases on average by one quarter just because of the visit to the doctor. Even talking increases it in virtually everyone. A family doctor who knew you wouldn't be fooled.

Routine tests are very often completely unnecessary. They are carried out, according to a recent Lancet editorial, 'just in case'. The editorial cites evidence that only six out of 630 hospital patients were diagnosed from routine blood and urine tests. Routine x-rays, thyroid tests, swab cultures for the newborn are among the tests that could be dropped.

Besides, there are 1400 different tests. Nineteen billion were performed in the US in 1987, 80 tests for each man, woman and child, at a cost of $100 billion. With all these tests, it is quite likely that something abnormal turns up even in the healthiest person. They are also expensive, and some are risky or painful because they are *invasive*, that means that they involve probing, penetrating or injecting material into the body. Invasive tests to avoid unless you are sure that they are necessary are:

- Tests that end in -oscopy (bronchoscopy, laparoscopy, cytoscopy, etc.) which involve inserting an optic tube into the lungs, abdomen, ureter, colon, etc.
- Tests that involve injection of a contrast dye into some part of the body for taking x-ray pictures of soft tissue (e.g., barium enema). They often involve injecting dye by means of a long tube inserted into the blood vessels to reach specific sites such as the heart or kidney (coronary angiography, renal angiography).
- Biopsies, in which small amounts of tissue are removed, sometimes by needle from deep within the body.
- Tests that involve withdrawal of body fluids by needle from joints (arthrocentesis), womb (amniocentesis), bone marrow (bone marrow aspiration) or spinal column (spinal tap).
- Tests that involve high dose x-radiation (see page 35).

How to avoid unnecessary and mistaken diagnosis

Go into Diagnosis with eyes open. Here are some basic guidelines to help you:

- Be sceptical about any diagnosis of illness or abnormality that you don't already feel, especially if the diagnosis is based on lab tests. In that case, ask for a repeat of any abnormal tests, if possible in another lab. But wait a while for your second test. Sometimes abnormal readings are correctly identified by the lab but are due to a passing phenomenon.
- Remember that diagnosis should clarify symptoms you have, not make you look for those you don't have.
- Rely on an experienced primary care physician, especially a family physician, whom you trust and who knows you, more than on strangers, however qualified they may be. Your primary care physician, if he is good, will carry out a series of tests when you are healthy so as to have a base line in case you are sick. He should ask for repeats of abnormal lab tests as a matter of course.
- If lab tests and diagnosis show that you have the *beginnings* of a health problem such as 'pre-diabetic' or 'mild hypertension' treat it as a warning. Seek treatment from alternative or holistic medicine. Nutritional, natural-preventive, traditional, herbal, homoeopathic and oriental treatments all work well at the early stages of diseases, whereas conventional medicine does not. The drugs prescribed for pre-diabetes, raised cholesterol or mild hypertension often carry more risk than benefit, and any lifestyle advice your doctor gives you will have been learnt from natural therapists anyway.
- Don't be afraid to request a second opinion if your doctor advises the more serious invasive tests on the basis of lab tests for a condition which you do not feel. Take the lab tests with you but respect the second-opinion doctor's wish to do his own.
- Keep minor symptoms to yourself. Unless symptoms are serious, unusual for you, persistent or possibly related to some serious disease in the history of your family or yourself, don't run straight off to get a diagnosis. For example treat a headache

which you feel is a tension headache with a hot bath, a rest, a massage; treat a sore throat with lemon and honey; treat insomnia with herb teas of chamomile, lemon balm, or valerian; treat an autumnal fever with fluids, rest and cold water compresses.

■ Don't be continually diagnosed because you are worried about having a disease but there are no signs of it. It can be a dangerous indulgence.

■ If you must undergo an invasive test such as a biopsy or catheterization ask that you be shown the results and discuss them before further medical steps are taken. Do not sign a consent form to 'other measures that may be necessary'. Only permit the test itself.

Annual check-ups and screening: the holistic view

In an ideal world your practitioner would know you reasonably well. He would be giving you occasional health advice and instruction on your diet and lifestyle, and at the same time give you a general once-over. He would know one or more alternative medical skills, or work with someone who does, so as to provide you with holistic total body maintenance. Alternative medicine gives real teeth to preventive measures. For example an acupuncturist will not just tell you to stop smoking, but will help to restore a healthier balance to your body and mind so that you gradually feel that cigarettes are superfluous.

The above scenario is rather unusual in today's world. Conventional modern medicine's equivalent of the general once-over is the annual check-up. This is encouraged by private medical plans, and often insisted upon by corporations. The real advantage of an annual check-up is that it gives you early warning of the build-up of chronic disease. However the disadvantage is that you may leave the check-up with prescriptions when you should have had instructions. For example you may be discovered to have mild raised blood pressure and raised blood cholesterol. You may be told to reduce fat and salt and given drugs such as diuretics, beta-blockers and blood cholesterol reducers. Even worse, you have now entered the illness category and anxieties take the joy from your life. The 1979 Canadian Task Force on Periodic Health Examination carried out a three year assessment of the annual check-up and concluded it was 'inefficient and potentially harmful' because it rarely detects serious disease and often creates worry and harmful medical treatment of the reasonably healthy.

Go to a check-up by all means. But follow the guidelines that I have just given on what to do with diagnosis. In particular if a disease is found in its early stages, such as the detection of raised blood pressure and cholesterol, seek real professional preventive advice from a good alternative or naturopathic practitioner rather than beginning a possibly lifelong consumption of harmful drugs.

The mass screening is like the annual check up, but it involves checking large numbers of people for a single specific disease. There used to be screening for lung cancer until it was realised that regular chest x-rays of millions of people caused more illness than it cured. Mass screening, that is, screening of the entire population, is a bad idea. A few people are helped. But for every case of a disease that is caught early there is a case of a disease that is treated when it would have got better by itself, and a case of a healthy person treated or biopsied because the screening test gave a wrong result. The net result is that a screened group of people is no more healthy, has no fewer diseases, has the same amount of hospitalization and the same death rate as an unscreened group. Several studies have shown that it just wastes money, creates anxiety and leads to unnecessary treatment. The mass screening of all women for cervical cancer, the so-called 'Pap' test, is a case in point. The tests were around ten per cent in error in the UK, and even more in the US, meaning that many women go through biopsies, or even have their wombs removed, unnecessarily. The National Health Service in the UK takes three to four million cervical smears per year, but it has had no impact on the disease.

When is screening useful? Screening is genuinely worth while when it is restricted to special high-risk groups, for example industrial workers being screened for special diseases, or drug addicts for AIDS. A new scheme that appears worthwhile is the x-ray examination of women for breast cancer: it has learnt from old mistakes. Only those of middle-age and above are called every three years, and in initial trials in the UK only 20 women in 1000 are referred for further examination. Of these, five will have the disease. Therefore not many healthy people will have to go through an unnecessary and worrisome second examination. Yet it is expected to reduce breast cancer deaths by one third. In this case the benefits certainly outweigh the risk.

What is the harm in diagnostic x-rays?

Half the population of the UK and eight out of ten in the US have diagnostic x-rays every year. This puts diagnostic x-rays in a category of its own, since if there are risks, even minor, they are affecting all of us.

X-rays are very high-frequency waves which have so much energy that they crash through living tissues like birdshot through a bush. The body absorbs a little of this radiation in proportion to the density of its tissues. In diagnosis the shadows of the absorbed x-rays are recorded on a special film. The old x-ray machinery produced a greater energy of radiation which was scattered more widely; today the equipment is more accurate and the films more sensitive. This permits better pictures, outlining soft tissue as well as bone, using less total radiation. Special diagnostic techniques which use x-rays include fluoroscopy, in which the x-ray shadow of the body is cast onto a kind of television screen, and the CAT scan in which an accurate moving beam of x-rays builds a three-dimensional picture, usually of the brain. Sometimes a contrast medium, such as barium or a dye, is injected into parts of the body to make them more opaque to x-rays.

X-radiation causes damage to the genetic apparatus by which cells duplicate themselves. The damage could manifest as cancer, or abnormalities and cancer in the next generation, and there could be hidden risks we know little about. The lower the dose, the less the risk, but there is no lowest dose below which x-rays are completely harmless. Every dose bears its risk, and an added problem is that each x-ray leaves an indelible mark: the effects accumulate.

The following is a table of the dose received in various examinations — and the consequences, compiled by the US Health Research Group.

Type of examination	Dose at skin for each film (millirads)	Equivalent dose to whole body (millirads)	Likely no. of deaths from each million examinations
Upper intestines	500	400–800	30–100
Bowels and lower intestines	600	300–700	25–80
Gall bladder	770	200–600	20–70
Spine	1200–1900	100–500	15–45
Stomach, kidney, bladder	770	100–200	5–25
Breasts	1500	100–200	5–20
Pelvis	500	100–200	5–20
Hip, upper leg	1036	50–150	5–20
Skull or shoulder	2–300	25–75	2–7
Chest	500	20–60	2–6
Dental (whole mouth)	1100	10–30	2–6

The US National Academy of Sciences has calculated that one barium examination of the intestines gives as much cancer risk as smoking five to twenty cigarettes daily for a year. Even a dentist who delivers a very low dose is putting you at risk whenever he x-rays your teeth. This dose is equivalent to smoking half a cigarette every day for a year. This is why the American Dental Association has warned that x-rays 'should not be used unless there is reasonable expectation of benefit to the health of the patient'. If this is the case with dental x-rays, how much more so for the rest?

If a contrast medium is used, for example iodine, dyes or barium, there are added risks and it may be uncomfortable. Patients have successfully sued Glaxo, a drug company, because they incurred a painful disease, arachnoiditis, as a result of a contrast medium injected into their spine during spinal x-rays.

Obviously x-radiation is not completely safe. Yet at times it can be a very valuable diagnostic tool which undoubtedly can save life and limb. The problem is overuse. When I took my six-year-old daughter to hospital after an awkward fall from a church wall the x-rays showed a simple fracture of her shin bone. No question: the x-ray was worth it. But then there was a series of regular visits to the hospital to check progress, and each time the orthopaedic surgeon refused even to look at her without another x-ray. Healing was normal, and the x-rays were less and less necessary – a reflex of a doctor who didn't trust his hands any more.

In the United States the Food and Drug Administration has calculated that at the very least one third of all medical radiation is unnecessary, and at least half of all skull x-rays.

How to avoid unnecessary radiation

Diagnosis is the identification of a health problem. If the diagnosis carries some cost to you, as do x-rays, it is common sense to weigh up this cost against how serious this health problem is or might become. Each case must be decided on its merits. For example if x-rays are used to look for broken bones or internal injuries then they are justified. Likewise if they are used to diagnose a suspected serious disease, for example a breast x-ray to check a lump. At the other extreme some x-rays give little or no benefit to your health and well-being. You can refuse them. These include:

- Routine dental examinations in the absence of specific problems.
- Precautionary examinations to protect the doctor against malpractice actions (which may account for some 30 per cent of all x-rays ordered in the US).
- Examinations to quieten you or your doctor's anxiety that there may be something there. These just-in-case procedures are usually placebos. Placebos should be harmless.
- Bureaucratic examinations for jobs, institutions or the army. A friend of mine was called up on reserve duty. He was asked to undergo a routine whole-body x-ray by the military doctor. 'What should I do?' he asked me, 'Is it really so bad? Why would the doctor ask me to do something against my health?' 'It is not a great risk,' I replied, ' but the risk is there nevertheless and it is a medical habit to ignore it. The question is, why should you accept any risk without benefit?' He refused the x-ray. The

doctor was somewhat taken aback but accepted instead a letter from his family physician that he was healthy.

Yet in most cases the benefit will be less clear than with a suspected fracture. You can clarify the situation by asking what question the x-ray is trying to answer, and what will be the consequence of not having an x-ray. Share your concern with the doctor that you only accept an x-ray if it is absolutely necessary.

Before agreeing to an x-ray, find out if there are previous ones that can be used. Around 30 per cent of dental x-rays repeat already existing films, and doctors sometimes find it more convenient to take new ones than call for films that may be in another hospital. So keep track of all your old films, especially if you move to another dentist or physician. Use the table on page 38 to help you. If an x-ray is necessary what can you do to minimize exposure?

- Make sure you wear a lead apron, even in dentistry. The most sensitive organs are the testes, the ovary, the thyroid in the neck and the thymus in the base of the neck. These must be covered.
- Obey instructions during the x-ray to avoid a retake.
- Check if the machine is a new low-dose type (these have rectangular apertures).
- Protect children, especially the unborn. Pregnant women should refuse x-rays unless a serious disease is suspected. As a precaution, all women of childbearing age should only be x-rayed during or just after menstruation. Young children are more vulnerable to the cancer-causing effects of x-rays, and as they are smaller, more of their bodies will be in the spreading path of the x-ray beam. Children will be parents. Make sure that they too are shielded, for example during dental x-rays.

Can I protect myself from x-rays?

X-rays damage the cells of the body by so charging up certain molecules that they 'go berserk'. These supercharged molecules are known technically as *free radicals*. Now the body already runs its own housekeeping system to remove any free radicals that may

Your radiation record

Keep track of your examinations and films

Name:				
Address:				
Date	Doctor and hospital	Type of x-ray	Dose	Where films kept

occasionally arise during the normal course of events. This damage-repair equipment includes vitamins C and E, selenium and sulphur-containing amino acids (protein's building-blocks) such as cysteine and glutathione. There is good evidence that these substances can protect against radiation. For example the organism with the highest level of these substances is a bacterium, radiodurans, which lives happily in nuclear reactors. Cysteine is the substance given in hospitals to people who have accidentally received a radiation overdose.

Soviet space researchers have tested some 25,000 different substances to find a radiation protective for their cosmonauts in space. They reasoned that an ounce of radiation protection inside the body of the cosmonaut is worth a few tons of shielding on the outside. The cocktail that emerged from their tests, which they gave to their cosmonauts, contained the amino acid cysteine, along with another one histidine, vitamin C and the bioflavonoids, B vitamins, and certain stimulating herbs, particularly ginseng. Vitamins B5 (riboflavin) and B2 are known to help protect against radiation.

Though there is much classical laboratory research on cells, tissues and laboratory animals, there is a lack of clinical research demonstrating that humans taking supplements of these house-keeping substances during diagnostic radiation are actually protected from damage. However it may be a sensible precaution to do so starting a few days before higher-dose x-rays such as the barium intestinal series or the CAT scan. A suggested anti-radiation cocktail would be as follows:

- 500 milligrams of natural vitamin C, three to four times a day.
- 100 to 200 micrograms of selenium a day. This can be taken in the form of selenium-yeast. High doses of selenium are toxic.
- 50 milligrams of vitamins B2 and B6 and 100 milligrams of B5 (pantothenic acid) per day.
- 250 milligrams of cysteine three to four times a day at the same time as the Vitamin C. This can be bought in some health shops. It may interfere with injected insulin so do not take it if you are diabetic. Cysteine is found in eggs. An egg contains 250 milligrams, more if it is from a free range hen. You could also eat onion and garlic which contain cysteine-like ingredients.

Chapter Three

HOSPITALS: KEEPING YOUR HEAD, KEEPING YOUR HEALTH

Sanctuary or factory?

Janet Marshall was seriously injured in a car accident. She was taken to a public hospital locally, and stayed there for six months. This is what she told me:

'There was a team of nurses on duty at my ward for 24 hours. They insisted on carrying out a very high standard of personal care for they said that morale is the basis of recovery. They bathed my feet and did pedicure frequently, even though I was paralyzed from the waist down. Every morning either the physiotherapist or the nurses themselves gave me a massage, sometimes using essential oils. Every other day all the patients had electro-acupuncture given by the physiotherapist to stimulate the nerves and tissues to repair the damage. Morning and evening they would give out hot moist bags which were enthusiastically welcomed by the patients who would place them on their body with a lot of fuss and discussion, and they would clamor for more and more. I also had water therapy for six months until I regained full use of my limbs. The most touching part was that every person, from the cleaners to the doctor, felt they were part of a team whose sole function was to get me better. There didn't seem to be favourite patients. The team worked with enthusiasm, and were sensitive to all my special needs. For example I felt at one stage that

I was going out of my mind, lying there for such a long time. So a doctor came who taught me breathing exercises and he gave me a meditation to carry out to open energy centres in the body.

I experienced some problems initially, when the doctors gave me strong drugs that seemed to fog my mind. The doctors couldn't understand my difficulty so they called an arbitrator who sorted it out. He was a doctor himself who had been a hospital patient and therefore could take the patient's part very effectively.'

You may have been reading Janet's account with more and more astonishment. It doesn't sound like any hospital that you know of. In fact it happened in Japan and the hospital concerned was the Red Cross Hospital in Kyoto. It may give you a glimpse of what a hospital could be.

We cannot expect a hospital to be the pleasure-dome of Kubla Kahn, yet we might reasonably expect a hospital to make us feel well, to heal and support us as well as carry out necessary repairs.

Yet, as we know, when we enter today's hospital seeking help we are immediately stripped of clothing, belongings, personality, freedom of action, of movement and sometimes even of speech, for there is no one to answer our questions. We have to cope with uncertain rules of 'good behaviour' on top of the discomforts of isolation, strangeness and helplessness. 'Good patients' are stoical, docile, uncomplaining, unquestioning and don't take up much of the doctors' time. Staff discourage patients from being communicative, alert, active and strong willed. Yet these are precisely the qualities needed for recovery, especially of long-stay patients.

It is especially hard on children. They feel the atmosphere of alienation, isolation and anxiety more than adults. The children are expected to behave like good adults in the same way that adult patients are expected to behave like good children.

Why is it that doctors are well known to be the most difficult patients of all? Mostly because lying in bed they are faced with their own creations. As Dr Jack Geiger described in his book *Humanizing Health Care*:

'I had to be hospitalized suddenly and urgently on my own ward. In the space of only an hour or two I went from apparent health and well-being to pain, disability and fear, and from staff to inmate in a total institution. At one moment I was a physician: elite, technically skilled, vested with authority, wielding power over others. The next moment I was a patient: dependent, anxious, sanctioned in illness only if I was cooperative. A protected dependency and the promise of effective technical help were mine – if I accepted a considerable degree of psychological and social servitude.'

The hospital environment can seem like a factory – with its fluorescent lights glaring on shiny pastel corridors and bleached faces. Instead of being restful, secure and unpolluted, hospitals are awash with noise, chemical and electrical pollution. The US Environmental Health Agency found that an average patient in a recovery room experienced noise equivalent to a car, and in the operating room the noise was equivalent to a diesel truck. The bright lights, chemical smells, electrical machinery added to drug side effects and anxiety create ideal conditions for headaches, migraines, rhinitis and reduced resistance. As one staff member complained in *The British Medical Journal* about his hospital: 'Ever since it opened there has been a high incidence of complaints of sore throats, nasal congestion, headaches and lethargy among staff.' And the patients?

All this was assumed to be a minor inconvenience, an inevitable price to pay for the miracle of modern medicine. However it is less acceptable now in the 1990s when we have become concerned with health, not only with saving lives. There is also a darker side to the hospital which we should be aware of. It is in the little known statistics of unnecessary operations (six million in the US causing perhaps 50,000 deaths), drug side effects (around one in five of hospital patients), new infections acquired while in hospital (one in ten of all patients), and mistakes in diagnosis (around one in seven of all patients).

You can't rebuild all the hospitals, but there is a great deal you can do to make sure you get only the correct treatment and pass through the hospital as quickly and comfortably as possible. Again the new insights of holistic medicine offer a great deal of help.

Avoiding unnecessary hospitalization

If you enter hospital as an emergency case you won't be reading this book anyway, and you can skip this section. But most admissions start in your doctor's office or clinic with something like: 'I want you to go for a checkup to Mr Jones (the Specialist) at the Cardiology Department of St. Peter's Hospital.' But you are not yesterday's meek patient who trots unquestioningly in the direction indicated. This statement should be the beginning of the dialogue not the end of it. You should be sure that the problem is serious enough or mysterious enough to warrant that consultation. The following questions might help to get you started:

'What exactly is my problem and why do you think I have got it at this time?'

'Why do you think I should see that kind of specialist?'

'Why do you recommend that particular specialist?'

'Can you give me any advice on how to look after myself so that the condition is stabilized or improved?'

'What will happen if I delay my visit to the specialist?'

'What will happen if I choose not to visit the specialist?'

For Tests:

'What tests are you recommending and what questions do you need to answer?'

'What are the risks or discomforts of the tests?'

'Are there any other ways to arrive at a diagnosis?'

'What will be the costs?'

If you feel comfortable about that consultation fix the date a little in the future. Tests are rarely so urgent that you cannot get prepared, and you have some homework to do first.

Before the consultation get to know something about your suspected condition. The best sources of information are health magazines, popular medical books, (see Appendix 1) or where relevant, self-help groups (see Appendix 2). Check possible diagnoses relating to your symptoms and kinds of treatment options. Check also whether there are natural self-care or alternative methods which are relevant. You may benefit from a consultation with a naturopath, acupuncturist or psychotherapist who could at the very least give you a completely different picture of the disease and its origins and may also help you if you choose hospital treatment. You do have a chance of avoiding all further medical intervention. Some cost at this stage could save you a good deal later on.

One more useful tip: prepare a record of your symptoms and the questions you want to ask the specialist. You will be faced with a busy specialist, behind a pile of papers, who may hardly look at you. You may be rationed to a few squeaks about your symptoms interrupted by the telephone. So have your questions ready.

Choosing a specialist, choosing a hospital

It can be an agonizing decision. My friend's daughter was injured with a complex fracture of the elbow and taken to the nearest hospital. He waited outside, hearing rumours that this was a rather bad hospital for orthopaedic surgery. One hundred miles away, someone tells him, is a city hospital in which the orthopaedic department is headed by a top class man. My friend is totally confused. Is the other place really so good, and this place really so bad? How can he take his daughter out? Is it worth a daily four hour drive? Yet couldn't a bungled operation cause a life-long problem? What would you do in this situation?

Your own doctor is the first address. If you enter hospital or a consultation with a specialist through him, the particular specialist is his choice. His answers to your questions should make it clear why he chose this particular specialist. You should always go for the best. This means a specialist who has a great deal of experience at this kind of problem or that kind of operation, who has a good reputation among medical people and who works in the hospital that is renowned for the treatment of that kind of condition. Where medical treatment is concerned all other considerations, such as how far away the hospital is, should be secondary, and you should make this clear to your doctor.

There may be many reasons why a doctor chooses a certain specialist, and not all of them may be in your direct interest. They may be old friends from medical school for example. You should discuss with your doctor why he chose this specialist, and if he is the most competent and experienced possible. In the US your physician may only have admitting privileges at certain hospitals, and he may even have to send a minimum number of patients to them to retain his facilities there. So you should bear in mind that he may have his own interest in sending you to a certain hospital.

If you are being treated under the National Health Service in the UK, you will not have a choice of specialist. However your doctor does have some freedom to choose the department of the hospital, and he should do this according to its reputation for this particular condition, which is often synonymous with the reputation of the specialist who heads it. In the US, or in private medicine, you should ask for one or two possible choices of specialist and consider them. In the US, ask if they are Board Certified, that is have taken certain tough examinations of their competence.

When you and your doctor choose a specialist, use your period of homework to endeavour to check on this decision. Self-care groups, friends (especially any who are in the medical or paramedical professions) and past patients are the best sources of information. Ask them what they have heard about the specialists in question. In the US you can call the local Medical Licensing Board to see if the specialists concerned are in any trouble or are involved in any litigation. If you receive reliable information which conflicts with that suggested by your doctor, then return to him to discuss it. In my friend's case, he correctly delayed surgery for two days, went to see his doctor, checked with friends and went to look at the city hospital. His daughter was moved there at his doctor's request the next day.

The choice of specialist or surgeon is the first consideration. The next is the hospital. The choice of hospital is especially important if you are a health service patient as you then have no right to treatment by the specialist himself, but may be treated by a junior doctor working under him. You might therefore want to assess the quality of the team and the institution, as well as its top man; however you can assume that if the top man is good, so will be his team.

Hospitals vary greatly. They may be large or small; a local community hospital with 50 beds or a giant regional medical centre with 1000 beds. They may be teaching or non-teaching, specialist (children's, maternity, eyes, accidents) or general, short-stay or long-stay, with emphasis on nursing care or on high tech-surgery. They vary in standards of care as well as type of professional expertise. In some hospitals there is a high turnover of staff, unnecessarily rigorous application of meaningless rules, a stricter hierarchy, more mystification and uncertainties for the patient, less personal nursing care, and a feeling that the hospital is such a total institution that nobody would notice if all the patients disappeared overnight. In other places the reverse is true, and patients find a pleasing combination of a well-oiled system that nevertheless allows plenty of personal contact and individual care by the staff. This is not just a matter of comfort. It is also a question of your recovery. A study of different hospitals within the Manchester region found that it took eleven days to recover from appendix removal in hospitals where the staff were grumpy and didn't stay for long, and an average of eight days where the atmosphere was better.

UK hospitals which have 'opted-out' and US hospitals which are corporate owned tend to be more profit-oriented. This means that they might carry out more unnecessary treatments and tests and offer less of the vital 'invisible' nursing care.

Go and see a prospective hospital. If you are a private patient in the UK, and in the United States, you can ask to be shown around. Come at lunchtime to look at the food. Check if there is lounge and lobby spaces that patients can use, and can receive visitors.

Assess the availability of telephone, if the television is disturbing, if there are windows that can be opened for fresh air, and that have a view, if there is light, fresh air, space around beds, lack of noise and smells, and above all a good atmosphere among the nurses and patients. The best source of information on this is from patients in the hospital itself. However you can gauge quite a bit from the manner of the administer in answering your questions, in the way the staff talk to the patients (curt, patronizing, superior, professional and distant, or relaxed, friendly, warm and easy going).

Ask about the range of skills available (hypnosis? psychologist/counsellor?), visiting rules, use of library, how long it takes for nurses to answer calls, whether the kitchen can accommodate special diets, especially vegetarian and health food diets, and how often the doctors go round.

There may be more than meets the eye. A dingy, somewhat old-fashioned hospital may hide superb staff care. An example of this is the Birmingham Accident Hospital in the UK. Here the medical staff are divided into teams, the members of which work together without pulling rank. The lowest nurse can pipe a protest to the highest specialist. The patient always has the same team. The theme of friendliness is encouraged, and even ambulance crews visit 'their' patients to chat to them. The recovery statistics are unparalleled. In contrast, a highly modern brightly lit and efficient looking hospital may hide a distant and highly commercial atmosphere in which non-essential services are kept to a minimum, and human contact is non-existent.

Some points to remember:

- Smaller community or 'cottage' hospitals are often friendlier, with less chance of giving you a new disease or complication than the big teaching hospitals. But their treatment of unusual or serious diseases such as cancer could be inadequate, and they may not be up-to-date. Consider them for routine, un-complicated and safe procedures in which your fast and good recovery is paramount.
- Large, teaching hospitals and medical centres are, by contrast, better where there is life-threatening or unusual conditions. They may offer more up-to-date treatments. On the other hand

you may get less personal care, you may get many more un-necessary tests, and you may be treated by a junior if your con-dition is uncomplicated and routine. There is also more chance in the large hospitals of incurring medical side effects and new diseases and infections.

■ Teaching hospitals are less personal than non-teaching hospitals, and you may well be treated by staff under training for routine procedures. They can be more expensive, and you may not wish to be used as a living visual aid at a bedside lesson.

■ Some hospitals have less waiting time for non-emergency surgery, the College of Health in London publishes this information.

■ You may want to look for hospitals which include some form of natural medicine in their repertoire. Certain hospitals now run visualization and relaxation classes, have nurses who practice therapeutic touch, and even employ reflexologists/massage therapists, acupuncturists and counsellors for their patients.

■ The atmosphere and quality of nursing care, and availability of physiotherapists, are as important in long hospital stays as the expertise of the doctors. The longer the expected stay, the more weight should be given to the caring compared to the high-tech facilities.

Seeing the specialist

The specialist will normally be far more technical and less approach-able than your family doctor, and he will not know you. It is doubly important therefore that you ask for information and the true picture as discussed on page 43. Informed and relevant questions will not normally be rejected. Here are the basic questions:

'What is the illness and why have I got it?'

'What are the treatment options? How do their results compare?'

'What will treatment or surgery do? What are the risks? What will be the physical and psychological consequences and how long will it take to be back on form?'

'What will happen if I say no? Will it reduce the quality of my future life more than the possible side effects of the treatment?'

'What will happen if I delay it?'

'What will be the costs of surgery, tests, hospital stay, anesthetist.' (If private.)

'How frequently do you do this procedure?'

'Will you be doing the procedure yourself, or will a junior be doing it under your supervision?'

Despite your previous preparations you may find yourself sitting opposite quite the wrong man. He may not answer your questions, you may have a strong feeling of mistrust about him, or you may find out afterwards that he does not have experience or reputation for dealing with your kind of health problem. In these cases you can try to change your specialist. This is an easy matter if you are paying him: you just leave (not forgetting to take your x-rays under your arm). It is more difficult to change your consultant under the UK's National Health Service where you must accept whoever you are assigned to, so your options are: to go private, to start again completely with another local physician (not advisable) or to go back to your doctor, convince him of your case, and enlist his help. He will often do so despite the fact that he may be put in a some-what embarrassing situation with the present surgeon/specialist by supporting your lack of faith in him.

Second opinions

A second opinion can be a godsend. An extensive study at the Cornell Medical Centre found that around 25 per cent of those who were recommended surgery were told on second opinion that they didn't need it. Most listened to this advice. If the procedure is at all serious, or if the answers to the questions do not completely satisfy you, or if search has uncovered less risky treatment options, you should have a second consultation as a matter of course. Disputes can be settled by a third opinion. However, don't do an automatic round of second or third opinions simply because you

are nervous of surgery but you cannot find fault in the chosen treatment method.

Many insurance companies will pay for a second opinion as it
often saves costly and unnecessary surgery. If the decision is very
difficult or serious a consultant may suggest a second opinion anyway under the NHS. In serious cases you should always ask your
specialist for this second opinion.

The second specialist to whom you refer should do all the
necessary tests except those that are hazardous, including x-rays,
which you should bring with you. The specialist should know you
want advice, not treatment, so he will give a detached picture. You
should not tell him the diagnosis and conclusion of the first
specialist. Don't choose a specialist for a second opinion who is
from the same practice or hospital as, or recommended by, the first
one.

In the US there is a toll-free, government-run referral service
called the Second Surgical Opinion Hotline. The number is 1-800-
638 6833 (in Maryland 800-492 6603). You can also order a
Department of Health and Human Services booklet entitled 'Thinking of Having Surgery?' from: Surgery, DHHS, 200 Independence
Avenue SW, Washington, DC. 20201.

What are your rights in hospital?

You should know at an early stage what your rights are in hospital.
It may even have a bearing on your choice of whether to go. In the
US the American Hospital Association now issue a Patients' Bills of
Rights as a result of consumer pressure. They often don't show
them to patients, and in such a case you should ask for one on
admission. It covers matters such as your right to be informed of
all procedures and to give specific consent, rights of privacy and
confidentiality, and standard of service and continuity of care.

In the UK there are various laws:

■ You have no right to a particular treatment. You cannot demand
   vitamins, or a new surgical technique you know of, you can only
   ask your doctor about it.

■ You have a right to leave hospital at any time unless you are mad, highly contagious or helpless and abandoned by family and friends. Be prepared for opposition, however, and you will be asked to sign a form releasing the hospital from their responsibility for you.

■ You must be asked for your consent to all treatments (see below, page 103) and you must be told of the risks involved. Patients must be told the truth about their health and treatment except under exceptional circumstances.

■ You can refuse treatments even if you will die thereby. But the hospital can ask you to go if you don't accept their treatment.

■ If you are incompetent to give consent, for example if you are unconscious, or drugged, doctors can carry out essential treatments.

■ You can refuse to be treated in the presence of students even in a teaching hospital.

■ You have no rights to receive visitors outside the times agreed by the hospital. (But the Health departments in the UK and US have recommended hospitals to allow parents to visit their children at all hours of the day or night.)

■ You have no right to see your medical record. But a friendly doctor may quote from it or let you see it if you request. I have known patients simply to take their own file from the trolley going round or from the tray on the desk.

■ You have a right to see the manufacturer's information about any drug you are taking. If you can't get it easily from the harassed nurse or sister, you or your friend should go to the medical library and look it up (see page 158).

Self-care in hospital

You have accepted and agreed on the treatment and you get a date to enter hospital. Should you just pack a toothbrush and go? The thought may have crossed your mind if you have been in this situation: Is there anything I can do to reduce the risks of infections, complications, side effects and mistakes? Can I pack any health aids besides fruit juice? Holistic medicine is a rich source of methods and approaches to keep you as healthy as possible in body, mind and soul. Practices and remedies derived from holistic and natural medicine can not only protect you in hospital but also hasten recovery after the procedure. They can be summarised in the following chart. Each of these complement the other. For example a good supportive companion will get you supplements and health food, and allay anxiety. Alternative therapies such as reflexology or hypnosis help your frame of mind as well as immunity and recovery. Of course hospitals ought to provide these aids to health and well-being: it would help their recovery statistics. But they will not do so at the present time because such methods are outside the current medical dogma. However it is not impossible that consumer pressure will, in the future, force some hospitals to become holistic caring centres.

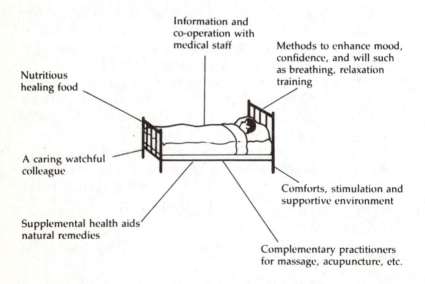

Information and co-operation with medical staff

Methods to enhance mood, confidence, and will such as breathing, relaxation training

Nutritious healing food

A caring watchful colleague

Supplemental health aids natural remedies

Comforts, stimulation and supportive environment

Complementary practitioners for massage, acupuncture, etc.

In the rest of this chapter some methods of holistic caring are discussed and outlined. In the next chapter we will concentrate on applying them specifically in the case of surgery, the most frequent treatment offered in hospital.

The Hospital Staff in the UK

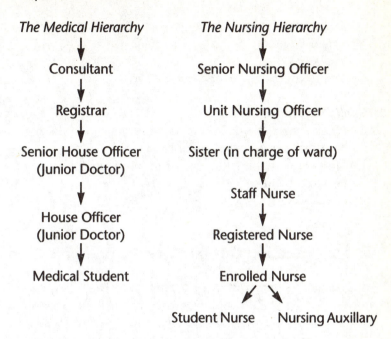

The Medical Hierarchy

Consultant

↓

Registrar

↓

Senior House Officer
(Junior Doctor)

↓

House Officer
(Junior Doctor)

↓

Medical Student

The Nursing Hierarchy

Senior Nursing Officer

↓

Unit Nursing Officer

↓

Sister (in charge of ward)

↓

Staff Nurse

↓

Registered Nurse

↓

Enrolled Nurse

↓   ↓

Student Nurse   Nursing Auxillary

Hospital Administrators
Clerical staff

Professional Staff – Speech therapists, occupational therapists and physiotherapists, dieticians, psychologists, radiographers, pharmacists, opticians, orthoptists etc.

Technical Workers – Biochemists, physicists, lab. technicians, dental technicians, medical photographers etc.

Ancillary Staff – porters, domestics, catering orderlies, engineers etc.

The Hospital Staff in the US
   Specialist
   Attending Physician (patient's own physician)
   Senior Resident
   Resident
   Intern (this category now rarely used)

The Nursing Staff in the US
   Nurse Care Co-ordinator (supervises nursing in the hospital)
   Nursing Supervisor or Senior Nurse
   Nurse Practitioners (can carry out more medical procedures)
   Registered Nurse
   Nurse Aids

Good protection through good communication

You are in the hands of the hospital staff. They can allay your anxieties or leave them to fester, they can make mistakes or get things spot on, they can disturb you and delay your recovery or care for you and hasten it. Your relationship with the staff is a key to good progress in hospital. For example full and proper information on what is going to happen to you can alleviate a great deal of stress and anxiety, and actually aid in your recovery. Nurses are, in fact, taught that good nursing care should include relieving the anxieties of patients so as to reduce complications during treatment. One of the main ways in which this can be done is to make sure you feel you are in control and involved in your treatment.

Staff are often very busy or tired, or they may feel it wouldn't help you to know more. Therefore you should insist in your pre-hospital consultation, and in hospital itself:

■ That you need full information on all aspects of your treatment.
■ That it will aid your recovery and increase your partnership in your treatment.
■ That you cannot give your consent without it.
■ That you are capable of understanding the information if it is presented to you in common language.

■ That this should be recorded in your notes so that other staff members and replacements know it.

This is easier than it sounds when you are faced by a brisk pre-occupied young nurse, or a curt superior doctor who looks as if he's permanently on his way to resuscitate somebody. So here are some tips on relating to staff.

Don't forget that hospital staff are human too, and may be receiving a daily dose of anxiety, alienation and institutional life for years on end. Nurses may start off as warm innocent young girls having to nurse bewildered, suffering adults. They are scorned if they show excessive feeling and sensitivity. They have to do what the doctors say, bear the brunt of their failures and receive no credit. Many nurses emerge as wonderful people in spite of it all. Try not to antagonize the nurses. Your doctor should receive your questions and, if necessary, complaints. Treat the nurses as your allies. That is what they are trained to be even if they are squeezed out of this role by doctors' power.

Talk to the nurses and doctors about themselves. Look them in the eyes. Ask why they are rushed. Find out what they are interested in. It is in your interest to be seen as an individual, as a person.

You want staff to see you as a good patient yet also a questioning and independent one. Be all the things they want you to be – cheerful, friendly, co-operative, considerate – except the grateful victim.

If you request things which are not done, if questions are not answered, first ask why. You can argue and complain but this very often fails with busy sisters and staff. Instead – just drop out. Refuse the medication. The doctor will come and you can tell him the problem on more equal grounds. If that doesn't work either, use an arbitrator, an intermediary. Your friend, an occupational therapist, the Patient's Representative (if there is one) or the hospital social worker can be called to your aid.

You can often avoid clashes, however, by preparing the staff just as they prepare you. Tell them from the beginning that you are a natural-minded person and against any and all drugs unless they are an absolute and essential part of the treatment. They won't know otherwise. Here is a case which illustrates what can be gained from this kind of approach:

Robert Mason, a 32-year-old cancer patient at a specialist cancer hospital told me how strongly he felt that it was extremely important to know all about his illness. He sensed that if he didn't know what was happening he couldn't help himself. He insisted on seeing the x-rays, talking to doctors – and taking and reading his case notes. The staff resented this; they only knew about it when he gave them back. But he persuaded them to support him by saying 'I have created my illness, I take responsibility for it and I know I will get better.' Although they thought him an oddball they were enlisted to prepare his special natural foods, to give him enemas, and to play his relaxation tapes for him. One day he found nursing staff members all silently relaxing in their staff room to the sound of one of his relaxation tapes, and from then on they were his allies.

Last, but not least, trust the staff. It will help you, and them, to relax. If you have accepted and chosen the treatment, if you have received the information you need, if you are aware of the risks and benefits, you've done all you can. Now let them do all they can in an atmosphere of encouragement and positivity.

A beautiful place

Something about your environment can depress you or lift your spirits, give you a sense of alienation and fatalism, or instill a force of life and hope. It is often quite unclear to a patient lying resigned, sleepless, fretful and sick that his surroundings are to blame. In one study carried out in several US hospitals, patients whose windows looked out over greenery were less depressed, needed less pain killers and recovered more quickly than a similar group who were looking out onto concrete walls.

In holistic terms, the pictures, the walls, the fresh air and an atmosphere of freedom rather than oppression are almost as important as drugs and drips. This is beginning to be recognised. A new report by the National Association of Health Authorities in the UK recognizes *that some kinds of non-clinical care can increase death and sickness and others can reduce them*. It confirms that putting long stay patients in shabby wards without stimulus hastens their deterioration. It recommends carpets and soft chairs, pictures and plants. Flexible ward routines would allow people to sleep and wake according to their own rhythms, and more privacy would improve dignity.

Hospitals don't need to be depressing places. A large new public hospital at Newport on the Isle of Wight is designed specifically to lift the spirits and instill well-being to patients. There is a conservatory at the end of every ward which looks out over beautiful gardens, inspired by the French painter Monet, inviting patients to meet their visitors by its fountains, water-lily pools and secret gardens. Instead of the usual vistas of pastel plaster there are natural materials – wood, wool, stone – with plants and water consciously placed for their healing power. The beds have personalised surroundings and patients wake in recovery rooms under attractive mobiles slowly turning.

Even little things can help. The x-ray waiting area in one rather old hospital in Oxford has been painted by art students to look like the inside of a conservatory. The creepers are winding their way all over the glass panes, the pots are lined up on old planks, the seedlings sprouting. There is much to look at. You forget your anxieties, forget that it is all just paint on a white wall.

What can *you* do to create a healing environment when in hospital?

If you can, try and arrange a room for yourself, so as to obtain some peace. Natural sleep and relaxation are essential to a speedy recovery. Yet hospitals are so full of commotion that this is often impossible. If you cannot beg or buy your way into your own room try at least to find a window seat, looking out on something to hold your interest, preferably nature. At the very least request your bed to be screened for periods to suit you.

Pictures, postcards, posters, your favourite artist; they can warm your heart. Ask your visitors to put them up near your bed, or even on the ward walls when no-one is looking. Children's wards have them, but it is mostly assumed that adults fare well on a diet of yellow paint.

The fluorescent lights are another problem, creating eyestrain and headaches and stopping proper rest and sleep during the day. Our first child, in hospital immediately after birth, seemed to be a model baby – attentive, quiet, relaxed, feeding well – except when

the nurse came in to change her. Then she became the model crying baby. We found later that it was the fluorescent lights which
the nurse switched on that made her yell. Obtain the co-operation
of your ward mates to keep them switched off, or ask the nurse to
give you an incandescent side light instead.

Natural ventilation is especially important while in hospital. Lack
of it keeps in all the toxic pollution from plastics, gases, pipes,
insulation and so on. Good ventilation helps to reduce the chance
of catching a disease from somewhere else in the hospital. More
than that, natural currents of air carry negative air ions (negative
charges on the particles of dust in the atmosphere). They make you
feel good. Positive air ions are spread by air conditioning and can
give you headaches, lethargy, nose and throat discharge, catarrh
and depression.

Ask the staff for the windows to be opened (if they do). Failing
that negative ions can be sprayed by air ionizers. You probably will
not be allowed to plug in an air ionizer next to your bed because
the staff will be afraid (unnecessarily) of interference with their
machines and monitors. Try and find a battery operated ionizer,
and just put it by your bed. It is silent. At a home for handicapped
children, a visiting doctor who had cured his respiratory problem
with air ions suggested that a large ionizer be installed. *A survey of
results after installation showed a marked improvement in children's
health and happiness, and as a bonus the staff did not succumb to so
many infections.* Ionizers have been tried in one or two hospitals
and found to relieve pain and improve rest and recovery of
burn patients. They are widely used in Soviet hospitals and clinics.
Studies with animals have shown that air ionizers can effectively
prevent the spread of viruses. They are recommended for use in
air-conditioned hospitals by many experts, including the Environmental Protection Agency in the USA, and Bart's Hospital's team
on Environmental Health in the UK.

A friend indeed

Friend, colleague, relative – you should make sure that somebody
is there. He or she has a vital role to play in protecting you and

aiding recovery. Much of the stress of hospitalization – the fears, the alienation, the disturbances, the lack of information, can be unloaded on to your companion. He or she can hear your grumbles, take your mind off your future, administer vitamins and medicines, get your special food, help you to wash, massage your feet and work with you on your breathing and relaxation exercises.

A companion can discuss things with the medical staff when you haven't the energy, and make sure you are getting the proper procedures. But what they should not do is issue instructions to staff in your name, as there is one thing medical professionals dislike more than the patient telling them what to do – and that is the patient's visitor telling them what to do. Also there may be good legal reasons why visitors shouldn't interfere with the nurses, or do jobs that they are supposed to do.

This caring companion will have work to do, and is not the same as a gaggle of visitors, chatting and exhausting you with partying at your bedside. The companion may need to fight your battles for you, and should, if possible, have the capacity for that task. You should arrange it all beforehand with the right person.

You should ask the doctor or the head nurse/sister in charge whether you can keep your companion with you beyond visiting hours. Use the excuse that you have an anxious, nervous disposition and you need this support to help you recover. The report of the National Association of Health Authorities on patient care advises that relatives should be allowed to sit with nervous patients as long as they like, especially before surgery. You should know that one of the usual reasons given for banning visitors – the danger of infection – is completely false unless the visitor has some unusual disease! In fact there are studies showing that a friend reduces patient anxiety, and this is especially the case with birth (see Chapter 8) which, with a friend to help, proceeds with less chance of a Caesarean and complications.

On no account leave your young child alone in hospital. There is no greater aid to your child's recovery than you, and no greater hindrance than the gaping hole created by your absence. Research has shown that separating young children from their mothers after surgery can increase the possibility of infection and haemorrhage. It may be hard on working parents, but leaving children alone does not save anything because children who are left in hospital regress and will certainly have their own back afterwards in terms of bed-wetting, crying at night and clinging or aggressive behaviour.

Most hospitals allow parents to be with their children all the time, but few have rooming-in facilities, or folding beds for parents to sleep by their children. However as the Patients Association comments: *the mother with an air-cushion, vacuum flask, knitting and determination can usually manage to sit up at night by the child's bed if she quietly makes up her mind to do so.* The Department of Health and Social Security in the UK, the National Institute of Mental Health, and the American Medical Association all strongly recommend that hospitals encourage parents to stay with their children. It is worth remembering this if you ever clash with staff about hospital visiting rules.

Stress and anxiety in hospital

You may feel you are going a bit crazy in hospital. But you will not be alone. Other patients feel the same although they may not talk about it. Research has shown that most people feel quite a lot of anxiety as soon as they enter hospital. This can even be measured by monitoring the alarm hormones (corticosteroids) circulating in the blood. These increase as soon as you walk through the door of the hospital and can stay high during your entire stay. Anxiety and disorientation during a hospital stay may be due to the strangeness, lack of information, the alienation, the lack of contact with the staff, the fear of painful or damaging treatments, being helpless, the demands to fit into the institution, or drug side effects. If you feel anxious or disturbed it might help you to pin this feeling down to causes such as these.

Stress and anxiety is a side effect of conventional medical treatment that is not taken seriously enough. It is largely the result of strong and even risky treatments being carried out on you by strangers in an inhuman environment. Anxiety in hospitals is known to delay recovery, and reduce sleep and appetite. Studies published in the nursing journals show how patient anxiety can increase the chances of infections and complications. For example a study on patients who had dental surgery found that if they were very anxious there was more tissue damage, which healed slowly. They also complained of more pain and had to be given added anaesthetic.

Here is another true example. June Pressman, a 30-year-old woman, entered hospital for an operation for an enlarged infected appendix. On the operating table surgeons found the abscess to be on the stomach wall itself rather than the appendix. They inserted a drain, but for three months the infection did not clear up, and caused her much discomfort. She says:

'I came to hospital on Thursday afternoon and tried to sleep early, as I was exhausted from worrying about my own health and about my mother who was completely dependent on me. Though ill, and in pain, I could hear the birds outside which made me cry as I felt cut off. I couldn't relax. They gave me a sleeping pill and eventually I dropped off but the next morning I was thick and woozy. The junior surgeon came to give me a few words and write up my notes, which was helpful, but the anaesthetist didn't visit me as he had promised even for the premed. The specialist came by and asked me how was the operation, which I hadn't yet had, and these confusions made me terribly tense and panicky. They wheeled me through a waiting area to the theatre, and the surgeon waved, but the theatre staff were very impersonal and clanked about like dustmen. The premed made me feel like a zombie and even more confused and as things weren't going according to plan I became terribly upset. I remember chewing my lips when they gave me the injection. I awoke in the recovery room crying and sobbing and after a few words with a gowned someone or other, I was wheeled back to my ward. I was drained, shattered, depressed and I wanted to die.'

Perhaps because of the stress her recovery was painful and prolonged. The infection didn't clear up and she was told she would have to come in again for another operation.

Clearly, the staff are usually too busy to be able to try to unburden you of your anxieties and fears. If you tell them, the usual answer may be more pills for you in the drugs trolley – tranquilizers and sedatives which are almost automatically issued to patients every evening. My wife was awakened from deep sleep after childbirth by a nurse who shook her and shouted 'Don't you want your sleeping pill, dear?' These drugs leave the original problem unsolved and add to it confusion and dullness, as well as some other side effects. They prevent you, inside the fog, from coping with the problem. Tranquilizers have also allowed the staff to continue their ignorance of the mental state of patients. Nurses know little; doctors less. You will have to help yourself. Here are some ideas.

Information

Jennifer Boore, Professor of Nursing at the University of Coleraine in Northern Ireland has written a short book on a sensitive study she carried out entitled: *'Prescription for Recovery'*. Forty patients about to undergo gall bladder and hernia operations were sympathetically prepared with information about the preoperative medication, the transfer to the theatre, the drips, anaesthetics, tubes and procedures, and the likely feelings and pain afterwards. Forty other patients having these operations had a general chat instead. The group who were fully forewarned were much less anxious and had less stress hormones in their blood. Only six out of 40 had an infection in their wounds or urinary system afterwards compared with 15 of the uninformed. At the fifth day after the operation those who had information began to shoot ahead physically and mentally. *It is the responsibility of the nursing practitioner*, concluded Professor Boore, *to ensure that such instruction is included in preoperative care of the surgical patient.* Tell it to your nurse!

Information takes away stress and anxieties by giving you the feeling that you are in control, that you are deciding things along with your doctor. This is particularly the case with surgery which is much more stressful than other treatments. A classic book on medical stress has described how proper information acts as 'psychological inoculation', which reduces the need for drugs and drips and hastens recovery. You should ask to know what you will feel, what will happen, what choices might have to be made, what the procedures are, and how long you will take to recover. This is in addition to the prior information you will already have obtained from the specialist and your own research which will have shown you the risks and benefits of this and other treatment options. For example, if surgeons would tell you that it might take you many months to recover fully all your capacities after a hysterectomy, you would be less likely to get depressed afterwards.

Reducing stress and aiding recovery with relaxation and imagery

One of the most well tried methods of reducing stress, tension and anxiety, is deep relaxation, which has now been taught to millions of people. There are several methods in use, all of which are designed to create a calm centre within you. There is now a great deal of scientific evidence that relaxation methods can lower blood pressure, and stress hormones, control psychosomatic problems and improve well-being. They are proven to be more effective than tranquilizers. This is discussed more fully in the next chapter.

Though relaxation methods are occasionally taught in health centres, they are almost never taught in hospitals where they are most needed. A few holistic-minded nurses have tried: One American nurse wrote that: 'Not long after I arrived I began an evening activity offering relaxation techniques integrating yoga stretches, deep breathing and guided imagery. Patients learned to envision their bodies relaxing and imagine themselves in a peaceful, safe place. They often fell asleep before their customary request for a sleeping pill, and in the morning the patients did not experience their usual medication hangovers.'

It is most effective when learnt properly and practiced daily for a week or two. Therefore you should learn the technique from a teacher, from tapes or classes, preferably before you go to hospital, to use when you are there. The basic method is as follows:

First, lie flat and comfortable, if possible without a pillow or
with only one. In the case of stomach or back problems it may
be more comfortable to bend the knees. At certain times each
day, when you know the ward is quiet, and there is likely to
be a pause in the endless bustle, you heal yourself. You turn
off the light shining in your eyes if you can, and begin to feel
the parts of your body. First the toes on the right foot, then
the sole and the heel, let them feel heavy, solid, quiet, and
relaxed. Then all the other parts of the right leg, then the left,
part by part. This way you relax each bit of you, gradually moving part by part from the tip of the toes to the top hair of the
head. Now feel the waves of relaxation move through your
body and out as you exhale and feel with every breath more
deeply relaxed. Enjoy the feeling. You are held up, supported,
and yet light and warm as if floating on water. You are calm
and relaxed, calm and relaxed.

Practice this before any unpleasant or stressful procedure or
experience, if there is pain, before sleep, or at any time. If you are
in a ward that seems like Clapham Junction or Grand Central
Station during the rush hour, sometimes it may be hard to practice
your relaxation training without help. Therefore bring a cassette
tape of progressive relaxation with you and a personal tape
recorder with headphones.

June Pressman, who had such a hard time during her first
operation, went to a psychotherapist when she knew she had to
have a second one.

'He told me that the illness is itself just a symptom, and that
we need to get to the bottom of it. He used hypnotherapy and
deep relaxation to go back to my childhood and through this
I realised that I was torn by guilt for being such a naughty and
ungrateful child. It came out in a great deal of anxiety and
nervous caring for my mother, now disabled, which made me
ill. We made a tape together which teaches me to enter a

deeply relaxing space where I can feel, and be comfortable with, all parts of myself. I am now confident enough to go back again for more surgery to remove damaged intestinal tissue.'

This time, armed with her tape and a personal cassette recorder, she is in charge. She has work to do. She is relaxed, ready for the treatment, understanding what is required of her and what the doctors have to do. She does not need to fight them either, for she knows she will be well, and she is.

Once you have learnt to relax properly you can use it as a starting point for various kinds of self-healing methods. You can give yourself affirmations, quiet verbal instructions to your body and mind, of the type recommended by Dr Ainslie Meares and Dr Ian Pearce, such as:

Relax, Relax, Relax,
Completely calm,
At peace, utterly at peace,
Feel this peace spreading through me,
In my face, in my body, in my mind and breath,
Breathing easily.
Relax, Relax, Relax,
Nature is at rest,
Relaxation renews strength,
Restores strength of mind and body,
Strength of body is in calmness of mind.

These affirmations can be general, or directed to particular organs or parts of the body in brief, energising 'conversations' with each part.

A variation of this method is autogenic training (AT) which should be learnt before going to hospital. It is an excellent psychological preparation for hospital, designed and taught by aware doctors. AT teaches people to enter and use the state of 'passive concentration' – the deeply relaxed yet aware state we have described by focusing on sensations of heaviness and warmth in the body. These are the stages:

1 Concentrate on the heaviness of each part of the body, for instance, 'My right arm is heavy'.
2 Concentrate on the warmth in each part of the body, for instance, 'My right arm is warm'.
3 Be aware of the heartbeat and feel its regularity: 'My heartbeat is calm'.
4 Be aware of the calm regularity of the breath, for instance, 'My breathing is calm and regular'.
5 Be aware of warmth in the abdominal area: 'My solar plexus is warm' (omit this exercise if there is an abdominal condition or bleeding from abdominal organs).
6 Be aware of coolness in the forehead: 'My forehead is cool'.
7 Come back to yourself with 'I am refreshed and alert.'

There are further series of affirmations which can be used to heal various parts of the body, which should be taught by an AT instructor a month before entry to hospital.

Once you know how to relax you can use images, which are powerful tools to heal yourself. You could start by using your imagination to arouse pleasant feelings in your body. For example you could imagine yourself being massaged over your whole body with warm oil, giving you a lovely warm feeling. After some time with this imagination you could imagine yourself massaged with light. Or you could imagine yourself on a beach hearing the sound of the ocean, smelling the fresh breeze and feeling the light and warmth of the sun on your body. Imagine that you are lying in the sand letting it run through your hands and feet.

It is useful to give permission and encouragement to the medical treatment you are receiving. Imagine the drugs spreading through your body and healing you. Imagine also your kidney and liver working to clean them out efficiently after they have done their job. Imagine the circulation cleaning and sweeping all the residues of disease. Think about the images which 'turn you on'. For example if you can get pleasurably lost in an English country garden when you smell real lavender, take a sachet into hospital with you and use it to help the images. After the war in the Lebanon healers were working in hospitals in the North of Israel with wounded soldiers. Each soldier received packages of pure aromatic herbs. One gravely wounded soldier would sniff it each time the pain became unbearable and cry out 'Hotel De Luxe'!

Imagery is a powerful process. One young man called Brian came out of surgery after an accident in a terrible state. He was screaming with pain, shocked and scared. He couldn't sleep for days because he was sure that he would die in his sleep. His friends brought in someone who knew him who had used imagery before. She quietly suggested that he walk in his own garden and guided him through it. He calmed down. Then she suggested that he give the body two hours rest. The next day when she came she found him cross with her. He told her he had slept, but why only two hours?! She then worked with images to clean his body and mind of the memories of injury and surgery and he was soon rapidly getting better.

You can work on images yourself, but it is always better to have some help in inducing the right image for you and your condition. For example one patient may be able to concentrate easily and precisely on a part of the body, and another might respond to a more general image of the 'walking by the sea' type. If you are lucky, your teacher for relaxation will be able to work with you on going to the next stage of guided imagery. If not, find a therapist, perhaps psychotherapist, nurse or counsellor, who knows the technique and can give you some instruction and make a tape to take with you.

Obtaining holistic therapy in hospital

You may well be asking: who on earth can I find in hospital that could help me with relaxation instruction, let alone massage and acupuncture? And as there is unlikely to be anyone in the hospital can I bring an outside acupuncturist to see me? Won't the staff throw him out on his ear?

Once you scratch the surface in the hospital, you will be surprised at the healing skills certain people have but don't advertise.

The people to look for are the paramedics – physiotherapists, occupational therapists, dietitians, art and music therapists and social workers. Some will have learnt alternative methods such as massage or counselling and will be happy to be invited to practice them. Occupational therapists may already know how to teach relaxation, which they use for rehabilitation, and guided imagery which they use for the confused elderly.

Normally the doctor decides if a patient needs the added help of a paramedic. However, ask the head nurse or sister (they are not the formidable starched white battleships they used to be). Your request will normally result in the paramedic popping in to see you. After that it's up to you. This is often the easiest way to obtain alternative treatment in hospital. If it is a doctor or nurse rather than paramedic who practices alternative therapy in the hospital, you can ask your doctor to arrange a meeting. However it would be better to arrange this with your specialist before you enter hospital – you are less likely to be able to organize it once in the ward. Furthermore you should meet with that staff member beforehand in case they are not suitable. For example you may hear there is an acupuncturist in hospital and you ask to see him for insomnia or drug side effects. However, like many medical acupuncturists, it may turn out that he only knows about pain and may not even admit the possibility that acupuncture can be useful for anything else.

You can request alternative therapists such as homoeopaths, acupuncturists, reflexologists and healers to visit you from the outside but you should ask permission of your specialist or doctor, preferably before admission. You should explain why you need the therapist in such a way that the specialist will understand. Don't say 'for my aura', as he'll reply 'oral what?'; say it's for anxiety, psychological support, or pain relief without drugs which you are sensitive to. If he thinks it will help you recover more quickly there is a 90 per cent chance that he will not object. After all he will get the credit for your successful recovery! Even a UK Department of Health brochure on patients' rights mentions that spiritual healers can visit patients in hospital. It will be somewhat easier if the alternative therapist you wish to bring in is medically qualified.

Where you encounter complete refusal to have an alternative

medical visit, you can usually disguise a healer, reflexologist, or hypnotist as a close friend or counsellor and get away with a surreptitious treatment behind the screen or under the bedclothes. This used to be the way, but thankfully, these days this is becoming less and less necessary.

Yoga in a hospital bed?

If you are set for a long period in bed there are certain consequences which you should be aware of. Immobility may cause wasting of muscles, loss of vitality, constipation, and the possibility of blood clots or sluggish circulation. It becomes more difficult to get rid of toxins due to drugs and poor digestion. All the pumps, vessels, and valves in the body slow down. Besides, lack of exercise can make you more vulnerable to the infectious agents lurking in hospitals: gentle yoga exercises can help to keep the lymph vessels pumping their protective fluid around the body.

Yoga is the best self-care method under these conditions. The word 'yoga' may conjure up visions of patients doing headstands on their beds all along the ward. However it has a gentler side. Stretching followed by deep relaxation is an excellent exercise which can be carried out in bed provided that new operation scars are not stretched. All the postures suggested below should be done very slowly and carefully, feeling your way into each new position, checking for any strain, pain or cramping. In such a case, always draw back in case you hurt yourself. Do it more gently. The key is gentle and frequent rather than arduous and occasional.

Start by stretching all of your body with your hands above your head if possible. As you stretch up, imagine you are tall and long, and that there is space between your hips and your torso. Imagine space between your joints. Then stretch one side and the other, and each of your limbs in turn. You can rotate the joints of arms, legs, and neck, describing circles with the feet and hands, again feeling the joints open and loose. Tensing and relaxing individual muscle groups throughout the body, including the perineal region (the crotch), is very helpful in getting the circulation going, lifting mood, muscle tone and general wellbeing. If you are sitting you

Some yoga postures that may be suitable for patients

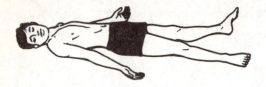

"Savasava" pose
for relaxation

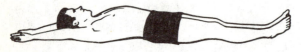

"Supine" pose

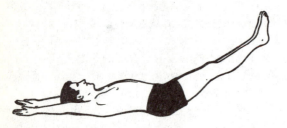

Alternate and both
leg "Leg raising"

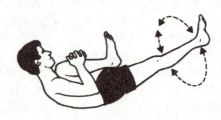

Alternate and
both leg "Wind
ejector"

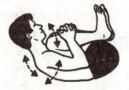

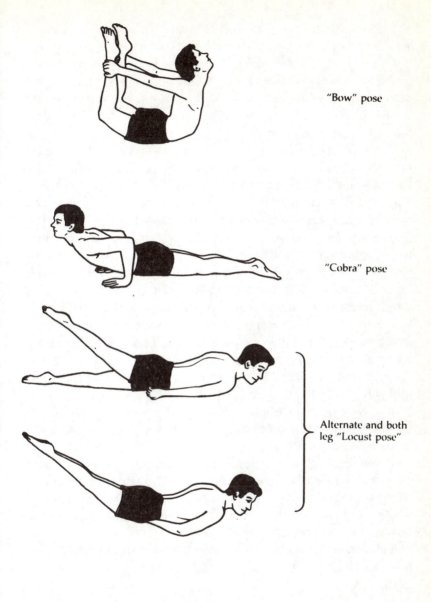

"Bow" pose

"Cobra" pose

Alternate and both
leg "Locust pose"

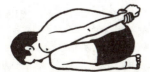

"Child pose"

can add twists of the trunk and sideways bending and swaying. You can do shoulder lifts, and describe circles with your arms. There are a range of specific postures and exercises for specific health problems which you should learn before you enter hospital from a competent yoga instructor. Some ideas are presented on pages 70–71. However care should be taken to make sure it will not interfere with your treatment.

Breathing methods are the main gift of yoga to the sick or recovering. Steady, slow breathing in the yoga fashion is one of the best of all methods for calming the mind and reducing tension and anxiety, and it acts fast. Within a couple of minutes of starting yoga breathing there are far fewer stress substances in the blood. The extra ventilation and oxygen gives energy, drives out accumulated toxins and drug hangovers and can lift depression. In yogic terms, steadying the breath steadies the mind and conserves energy. It helps to create a uniform flow of 'life force' (*prana*) in the body, which restores disturbed organs. In addition yogic breathing helps to create a relaxed awareness which can dissipate fears, conflicts and anxieties. Physiotherapists sometimes teach deep breathing after operations to help start up sluggish anaesthetised organs and prevent lung problems. But all patients in hospital would benefit, and you don't need the physiotherapist.

In a survey of cancer patients who used yoga, carried out by Dr Robin Monro in Cambridge, half said that yoga helped them to avoid tranquilizers and other pills, half said it helped avoid pain, while all of them stated that they had a more positive attitude to their disease and treatment. *The cleansing breath on recovery immediately after the head operation expelled the anaesthetic,* wrote one woman, *then, alternate nostril breathing helped to balance my emotions and induced sleep.*

A classical calming breath involves slow regular breathing with the exhalation steady and controlled and twice as long as the inhalation.

- Take a long even breath, expanding chest and stomach.
- Hold it for one and a half times as long.
- Exhale steadily, controlling the passage of the breath by restricting it in the throat, for twice as long as the inhalation.

- Try it with both nostrils at once, then each in turn.
- Concentrate on the feeling of the breath going in, the suspension when you retain it, and the release and out-flow.

A more energising, arousing breath makes use of the diaphragm:

- Inhale steadily, slowly and completely by expanding the abdomen so that it bulges a little. Let the breath fill the body like water filling a bottle. Then hold the breath for a moment, exhale smoothly by drawing in the belly and hold the breath out for a moment. Smoothly begin again.

Breath and movement can be combined with great benefit, but you should check with the medical staff or yoga teacher before exercises of this kind in case it is unwise in your medical condition:

- Raise the right leg slowly while breathing in.
- Hold the breath and the leg.
- Before any strain is felt, lower the leg and exhale, slowly.
- Do this with each leg in turn, with both legs, and with each arm in turn and both arms.
- Turn over if you can and raise your legs and arms in turn as before, while lying on your stomach.
- Start once or twice and build up gradually day by day.

Hospital food and nutrition

Beata Bishop, in her book *A Time To Heal*, recalls how she asked her doctor in hospital if he could recommend a diet to help fight her cancer. *The doctor shook his head. 'Diet has nothing to do with cancer. Just make sure that you eat plenty of good nourishing food to build up your strength. That's all.'*
   'Do you realise how abysmal the food is in this hospital?'
   'Oh, I've seen worse. And you won't be here all that long.'
   This sums up the official position on hospital food: you'll survive it. But will you?

Half the patients in general wards in the US and around one third in the UK suffer from malnutrition. Some may have come into hospital already malnourished. However the hospital food is also to blame. Even the *British Medical Journal* has complained about it, mentioning that people hospitalized for more than two weeks can become run down from poor food. Research has shown that in one of the top hospitals in the country, one quarter of the patients were found to be undernourished, and many received less iron and vitamins than the international recommendations for the healthy, let alone the sick. According to research studies, some hospital meals are so impoverished that you would have to eat two of them each time just to get the minimum requirements of minerals such as magnesium and zinc, and vitamins such as C and D.

The sad fact is that while hospital food may give you less than a healthy person needs, a hospital patient requires much more. Drugs destroy vitamins, stress uses them up, and antibiotics can prevent them being absorbed in the diet. At the same time larger quantities of vitamins such as vitamin C, and minerals such as zinc, are needed to ensure proper healing of surgical wounds and to protect you from infections and complications. A study of 500 patients in New Jersey hospitals showed that those with low blood protein from poor diet were four times more likely to have complications.

The research is clear – poorly nourished patients in US hospitals stayed in hospital for more than 15 days compared to ten days for properly nourished patients. An average hospital stay cost around $5000 for normally nourished, but around $15,000 for the malnourished, mostly because of infections, complications and slow recovery.

A hospital is the very place where you should have the healthiest meals of your life. Yet this was the food that met Beata Bishop on her arrival in a London hospital for cancer treatment: *Thin tinned soup, thin leathery meat, drowned vegetables, sliced white bread, tinned 'plastic' fruit compote, the kind of detestable food that left one both bloated and hungry...food that smacked of a third rate seaside cafe.* Although the food may be a little better today, hospital food has to be prepared in large quantities at low cost. So out go taste, balance, freshness. In come processed, refined, dehydrated and preserved foods. Unfortunately, medical staff are rarely interested in optimum nutrition, only in minimum nutrition.

How to get natural food in hospital

Fortunately the problem of hospital food is easy to rectify because you can get food brought in. However first you need to know what is available. The first step is to write to the administrator before-hand mentioning any special diets such as vegetarianism, and requesting unprocessed, additive-free, natural foods. Then see what comes. Some hospitals already offer concessions towards health foods such as brown rice or brown bread. If you receive reasonably healthy special meals, then all you may need to bring in is supplements (see below).

On the other hand if your first meal comes out of a tin, you should either abandon hospital food altogether and get your meals brought in, or pursue the matter by requesting to see the dietitian. Her job is to design diets for patients with special problems, such as liquid meals for those after stomach surgery. Ask the dietitian first about the hospital food – how fresh it is, whether the vitamins like B, E, C, and minerals like iron and zinc, are sufficient, and how many additives and preservatives it contains. This will help you to assess the meals. Then ask her if there are any special vitamin requirements because of the drugs you are taking. Then discuss with her your wish for nutritious natural wholefoods.

The dietitian is used to persuading patients, who are in hospital because of a lifelong diet of hamburgers, to eat some salads. You will be putting the shoe on the other foot. She may agree with you and complain that the medical staff don't care about nutrition and the kitchens get no money and the patients wouldn't want natural food anyway. Or she may be unsympathetic, reprimanding you for believing magazine articles. Most likely she will be able to arrange with the kitchen to give you a special diet, or at least a salad at the expense of the pudding. Cancer patients at University College Hospital and the Royal Marsden, for example, have been helped by dietitians to receive vegetable juices and a special natural diet.

The alternative of having your food brought in is, however,

preferable if your caring companion or relatives can organize it. You can at least get what you want. I knew someone under treatment with chemotherapeutic drugs who couldn't eat anything the hospital brought her and grew weaker. Her daughter discovered the one thing she could take: fruit salad. She brought it four times a day subtly laced with wheatgerm, walnuts, sunflower seeds and sesame seeds, with soya milk poured on top. This was her diet – and in the circumstances it was excellent.

In India, the families of hospital patients see it as their main duty to bring home-cooked food in little caddies. India is a culture where the health-promoting aspects of food are very well understood. It is quite clear that each person has a requirement for particular foods according to his state of health and his constitution. Therefore only the family, who know him, can be relied upon to design recovery diets. The same thing applies in the Far East. According to Janet Marshall all the wards in her Japanese hospital have little kitchens especially for visitors to prepare food they bring for patients.

Which foods in hospital?

Your diet in hospital should consist of light, highly nutritious food, with plenty of vitamins and minerals. Since you may not feel like eating a lot, each ounce should count. The keys to healthy eating in hospital can be summed up by five rules:

Avoid empty calories
That is, food that is refined to remove its extra fibres, vitamins, minerals and natural plant constituents. This is especially important if you only eat small amounts. Thus white flour, instant mashed potato, refined cooking oil, sugar, sweets, custard powder, are all empty, while wholewheat flour, whole vegetables, unrefined or cold-pressed oils and fruit are the corresponding whole foods. Professor Bender calculated, in a *British Medical Journal* editorial on hospital food, that patients can be forced to obtain all their essential vitamins and minerals from one third of their diet. The rest is just empty calories. Stodge is the old-fashioned word.

Avoid tinned, overcooked or preserved foods
Get hold of a fresh apple, don't have the tinned stewed apple. Get fresh peas, don't have those things that seemed to have been peas. They too have been emptied of nutrients by preserving and over-cooking. You need 'live' food to help you live.

Avoid ancient relics
A lettuce should taste like one and be fresh, otherwise the salad, which may be your main meal, will fill you up and give you little. Ideally, food should be grown organically and brought straight to you. An orange can lose 80 per cent of its vitamin C on storage, and chemically grown food has less nutrients than organically grown food.

Avoid chemical cocktails
You cannot taste the preservatives, additives, colouring and flavour-ing agents, but you can probably guess that the bright red jelly in front of you has never seen a real strawberry. Mass catered hospital food tends to have a lot of these additives. They add to the load of toxins, such as drugs, that your body may be struggling to remove.

Avoid fatty animal foods
There is no need to become a vegetarian in hospital. Yet animal fats displace the essential and health-giving oils from your body, and also hold a lot of the toxins of factory farmed stock. So eat lean and light meat if at all.

Rely on natural wholesome, unprocessed foods. For example:

- **Protein foods:** soya, lentils, sesame, chickpeas, free-range eggs, goat's or sheep's yoghurt and cheese, fish, tahini, nuts, tofu.
- **Carbohydrate foods:** porridge oats, wholewheat (not just 'brown') bread, root vegetables (especially sweet potatoes), brown rice, millet or buckwheat.
- **Fibre/vitamin foods:** salads, fresh fruit, dark green and yellow vegetables, sprouts, herbs, garlic and onion.
- **Fats:** cold-pressed oils, tahini, avocado, nuts, sunflower seeds, goat or sheep cheeses.

It is very helpful to eat a good nutritious diet before you enter hospital. Your immune system will be delighted. Then, during a short hospital stay you should eat lightly, choosing protein and vitamin/fibre foods rather than a lot of starchy food. You don't need the calories while lying in bed, and the extra bread or potatoes and particularly sweets will be a stress on the system which makes you tired and depresses your immunity.

It is also known that the performance of some of your white blood cells is reduced by saturated fats. Therefore take oils rather than fat or margarine, and if you can get cold-pressed oils so much the better – they contain more of the essential fatty acids that might well be missing from a hospital diet. Above all avoid foods deep fried in old oil or fat – no chips!

Drugs (especially antibiotics), immobility, surgery and a change of diet can play havoc with your digestion. Intestinal movement slows down, appetite is lost, nausea, gas, indigestion and constipation are common in hospital leading to more drugs. Quite drastic changes happen to the normal bacteria living in your intestines. They become invaded by unfriendly species. These species create irritations and food allergies, and they can lead to depression, headache, lethargy, slow recovery. There is research demonstrating that if the intestines are working poorly and invaded by the wrong bacteria, patients suffer from more infections and complications after surgery.

The natural bacteria are encouraged by vegetable fibre in the diet and discouraged by meat products and saturated fats. The vegetable fibre should come from salads and fruit rather than wheat bran which is concentrated and may be an irritant. It is advisable to get fresh salads and fruit that are organically grown, to get the full complement of vitamins and minerals. They can be juiced. Commercial fruit juices are not a substitute (see below).

As has already been observed, you may not eat and drink a great deal in hospital so what you *do* take in should be impeccable. Water from the tap is not. For example fluorine in tap water can delay healing of bones and tissues, according to one study, especially if it is combined with fluorine in toothpaste and as a contaminant in foods. Obtain bottled mineral or spring water. Make sure it gives the source on the label. Mineral water is widely used in Europe and in the Soviet Union as a specific treatment of various conditions such as arthritis, hepatitis, gastritis and bronchitis. A good mineral water can give you extra calcium and magnesium, selenium and iron.

Special foods for resistance and recovery

It may be invaluable to obtain concentrated highly nutritious food if you cannot or will not eat full meals. Here are some suggestions.

Natural live yoghurt
When made from goats' milk this is an excellent source of protein and will preserve your intestines against drug side effects. Try to have live yoghurt even in smallish amounts three times a day, (unless you are on Monoamine Oxidase (MAO) – inhibiting types of antidepressant drugs). If your digestion is already affected by antibiotics and dietary change, take tablets of Lactobacillus acidophilus, bifidobacteria or probiotic mixtures of beneficial bacteria, instead of laxatives, antacids and so on. These supplements are now readily available in health shops. They help to repopulate the intestine with its regular ecology of bacteria, and thus to restore digestive and metabolic health.

There is evidence that taking Lactobacillus acidophilus increases general immunity and prevents infections, adds to vitamin production, and improves general health. Curiously, farmers have long known that they can improve the growth and health of domestic animals by giving Lactobacillus. Such good husbandry would be welcome in hospitals.

Fresh vegetables and fruit juices
Get a friend with a juicer to keep a relay of fresh juices arriving at your bedside. Green vegetables, sprouts, onions, parsley, and carrots contain most of the vitamins you need. Juicing extracts them without the destructive process of cooking. Juices are essential to those on liquid diets. Freshly made juices are by no means the same as canned, bottled or boxed juices to which they bear the same relation as trees to paper.

Onions and garlic
These are key vegetables on the recovery menu. They are full of
special minerals and vitamins. They help in detoxification of drugs
and chemicals, stimulating the liver and urinary system. Garlic is
the queen of the preventive remedies as it is the strongest and best
natural antibiotic known for household use. It has been found
effective against very diverse germs including those resistant to
modern antibiotics, and nearly 100 studies going back to Louis
Pasteur himself testify to its effect in preventing and curing
infections.

It is best to eat garlic fresh, but it must be crushed. A good preventive dose is one clove three times a day. It can be made more
palatable by eating it with salad (especially parsley) or fruit. Fresh
garlic can be eaten without harm unless there is damage or surgery
to the mouth or digestive system, when you will find it too
pungent to take. In such a case you can take tablets of dried garlic which are without pungency, and almost without odour. However avoid deodorized garlic which is not of proven effectiveness.
You may be understandably concerned about the aroma, not wish-
ing to keep the medical staff away along with the vampires. I would
venture that the smell is a necessary and very marginal side effect
of your own medicine. It might even bring some light relief into
the tedious, pervasive smells of lysol and plastics. Garlic does thin
the blood, so it is not advisable to take it on the day of surgery or
where there is risk of haemorrhage.

Miso soup
One of the best recovery diets you can find is macrobiotic. This
Japanese diet involves a fine balance of food factors which can be
designed according to your particular condition. Miso soup is the
doyen of macrobiotic cooking, made from miso (fermented soya
bean paste), spring onions and dried vegetables, and sometimes
brown rice paste. There is nothing better. It is what I have after any
illness, to recover strength rapidly.

Chicken soup
The main thing linking Jews and Chinese is a great respect for
chicken soup. If you can get hold of the Chinese version from

Chinese or Japanese shops it can contain Royal Jelly or Chinese tonic herbs. It is a powerful restorative but should have bones cooked in it in the traditional way.

Cider vinegar
This is an age-old preventive remedy. Combined with honey it helps to prevent infections in the mouth, throat and digestive tract. Cider vinegar is a good douche or rinse against infections anywhere in the body. You can drink cider vinegar and honey as a tasty drink that will help your resistance.

Tofu, or bean curd
This is concentrated coagulated soya bean extract. It is easy to digest, pure, full of protein, and can easily be combined with other dishes. You can use it like cheese.

Vitamins and supplements: what to pack in your hospital kit

After all that we have said about food, why should anyone need to take vitamins? The main reason, of course, is that it is not always easy to obtain all the foods that you want in sufficient quantity. Extra vitamins are your insurance in case, despite nutritional efforts, your diet doesn't prove sufficient. Besides, certain vitamins have therapeutic effects in doses much too large to get in the diet: They are especially needed in hospital in order to:

- **Detoxify** the body and clean it of drug residues, anaesthetics or wastes from poor digestion. The B vitamins help by activating the liver and metabolism. Vitamins C, E and selenium help directly to burn up the poisons.
- **Prevent debility,** tiredness and in the elderly premature senility, which is sometimes due to a lack of B vitamins. Topping up with B vitamins stabilizes blood sugar and can increase energy and vitality.
- **Resist infections and hasten healing and recovery.** Even small deficiencies in vitamin C in white blood cells inhibit the

immunity. A lack of zinc inhibits the function of the thymus gland, which pours out cells that defend the body. Supplements of vitamin C, A, E, various B vitamins, zinc, and calcium/magnesium are necessary when resistance is lowered by a stay in hospital. For this purpose supplements should be taken two weeks before entering hospital.

■ **Help wound healing** and recovery from surgery. Vitamin C, E, pantothenic acid, B6 and zinc all help to knit damaged tissues.

■ **Increase absorption, digestion and metabolism of food.** If you are only eating small amounts, vitamin supplements are essential to make full use of what you do eat. For example extra vitamin C can increase absorption of iron by several times.

■ **Prevent bone and muscle weakness** and damage from insufficient movement and sunlight. Lack of exercise leaches calcium from the bones and they become weaker. Lack of sunlight reduces vitamin D levels, as do antacids, barbiturates, laxatives and other drugs. Vitamin D and magnesium control the amount of calcium absorbed and incorporated in the bones. The elderly in one old-age home in Boston were found, during winter, to absorb only one quarter of the amount of calcium in the diet because of a lack of sunlight and vitamins. Vitamin D, calcium and magnesium are required if in bed for some weeks.

Therefore, your basic hospital kit should contain on average:

Vitamin C: Two grams per day starting before hospitalization. It should be combined with bioflavonoids.
B Complex: B3 and pantothenate at around 50 to 100 mg each day and the others pro-rata. A high-dose commercial B-complex formula should be sufficient. Start before hospitalization.
Vitamin E: 300 International Units (IU) day. But do not take vitamin E on the day of an operation, nor if you are receiving insulin. Start before hospitalization.
Zinc: 20 milligrams.

In some situations you will need to add further supplements:
If you are in hospital for some time, and your diet is poor in nuts, seeds, milk products and seafood, add two grams of calcium and

20 milligrams of magnesium per day as supplements. Plenty of vegetables can replace the magnesium. Also, add vitamin D at 1000 IU per day if you do not have fish, egg yolks, or other vitamin D sources.

GLA, Gamma Linoleic Acid, is a specific essential fatty acid that acts as a building block for certain local hormones called prostaglandins. These hormones regulate immunity 'in the field', like lieutenants. Supplemental GLA, which can be bought in the form of evening primrose oil or blackcurrant seed oil, can support immunity and general wellbeing, especially if the diet contains saturated, old and questionable fats or oils.

The above recommendations are an average. If you wish to take supplementation more seriously I would recommend seeing an holistic practitioner or a naturopath before hospitalization who can design a regime specifically for you. It becomes more important to do so the longer you are in hospital. If in long-term institutional care you should ask a holistic practitioner for a nutritional assessment. This is a blood test which can detect obvious deficiencies of vitamins and minerals. A supplement regime can then be built to remove your deficiencies.

Massage and essential oils to bring life and energy

All through Eastern countries – travelling on Indian trains, in the Thai markets, in a multitude of Japanese clinics, you will see massage. Mothers to children, husbands and wives to each other and children among themselves. And you will find as much massage in hospitals as you will in the homes.

Massage is more than a pleasure to a hospital patient in bed. It can make a great deal of difference to the way the lymph removes toxic wastes, the way the blood circulates, the movement of sluggish organs and the efficiency of passageways in the body slowed by drugs. And, of course, it also helps immobile limbs with their tension, cramp and muscle weakness.

Massage for removing wastes and achieving these physiological results should be carried out by a trained masseur. One powerful technique that can be used is shiatsu, or Japanese pressure-point massage. This involves prolonged pressure on acupuncture points around the body. It can achieve the relief of specific symptoms as well as to generally awaken and tone up body systems, and keep body and soul together (this is not as flippant as it sounds, for in long-term institutions the 'soul', 'spirit' or 'life-energy' seems to just pack up and go, leading to lifelessness, lethargy and inertia). For example it can stimulate the appetite using the 'An-min' point outside the top joint of the little finger, stimulate the circulation on the opposite side of the little finger at the 'El-mu' point, and treat constipation and diarrhoea, headache, insomnia, tiredness, pain or nausea, all symptoms that may crop up as a result of lying in hospital beds under drug treatment. However you need to learn the skill for yourself or ask for a skilled shiatsu practitioner.

Reflexology is quite similar to shiatsu and perhaps more commonly available. An experienced reflexologist can treat these same problems by working intensively on special points and regions in the feet and hands. Massage therapists who work in conventional (sometimes called 'Swedish') massage will be more suitable for giving a general health and life-giving massage than working on specific symptoms.

This does not mean that you cannot massage yourself. Massage of the head and limbs is valuable when you are in bed, at the least because it keeps you active and in touch with yourself. It gives you energy and confidence. Here are a few tips:

- Massage the soles of your feet with your thumbs in a rhythmic way, with deep pressure and rotation, especially along the midline and the arch.
- Do the same on the palms of the hands and the base of the fingers.
- A fatigue point is on the middle of the top joint of the little finger and at the top of the nape of the neck: use rhythmic pressure.
- Pain points are on the ankles below and behind the ankle bone and in the joint between thumb and forefinger: use rhythmic pressure.

■ Help insomnia by firm stroking of the neck muscles and the lobe of the ear.
■ Massage your limbs slowly with long firm strokes, with concentration, for an hour a day.

Essential oils are powerful concentrates of herbs and can be used with massage, or you can just smell them. Most can be taken internally too, at no more than two drops four times a day. However as a few oils are not safe to take in this way, only do so under advice of an aromatherapist. Don't put oil into the eyes or orifices where it could burn, and check with small quantities first in case of a rare allergic skin reaction. Here is a table of safe and suitable oils and their uses:

Oil	Function
Rosemary or Ambergris	Restores circulation to tissues
	Relaxes tense muscles
	Useful for early bedsores
Basil	Lifts mood and awakens
Balm	Helpful for insomnia
Catnip	Helpful for insomnia
Comfrey	Helps healing, soothes irritations and bedsores
Wheat Germ	Massage over scars, irritations
Lavender	Antiseptic and cleansing oil
Peppermint	Aids digestion and loosens tension

Essential oils, the essence of many profoundly useful health-giving herbs, should, ideally, be provided in hospital as an alternative to drugs, for insomnia, digestive problems, and especially to lift mood. The Institute of Nursing has recently initiated an Aromatherapy Nursing Project at the Radcliffe Infirmary in Oxford in which female patients are given essential oils after surgery. First results are awaited.

Herbal remedies for bedsores and other problems

Herbs and natural remedies are *your* medicines, they are available for you to find, try, prepare and use, and they can be your answer to a range of distressing health problems that may crop up while you are in hospital. Some herbs are effective where conventional drugs do not work well, for example in skin problems. They are milder and safer, for instance, in the treatment of headache, insomnia or constipation. You should mention to your doctor any herbs that you are taking as pills or capsules. However herbs can often be taken in the form of teas (brought in a thermos by your companion), and used in place of the hospital's coffee and cocoa.

Bedsores

These are a result of lack of movement, pressure and lack of circulation in the peripheral areas of the body. They are not an inescapable part of long stays in hospital, as they can be prevented by excellent nursing, massage and exercise, and a balanced nutritious high-protein diet. If you are at risk of developing bedsores, make sure you take vitamin E supplements and B vitamins which help to utilize the high-protein diet that is part of the treatment. Try to avoid all hard fats, butter and margarine, and stick to the cold-pressed vegetable oils mentioned above. Also, take GLA (Gamma Linoleic Acid) capsules daily.

For preventing and halting bedsores, you have three options. The best is aloe vera gel. It helps to keep the skin moist and soft, and has powerful anti-infective and anti-inflammatory actions. You can buy it as a lotion or salve and rub it on. Vitamin E-enriched wheat germ oil can be bought in capsules which should be pierced and spread. It is anti-inflammatory, encourages circulation and enriches the skin. A third option is rosemary oil, in a lotion. It also encourages circulation in the periphery and like vitamin E, is an anti-oxidant. These preparations should be applied three or four times a day.

For the actual treatment of bedsores, the classical herbs are: astringents, especially witch hazel; mucilaginous agents which moisten and stimulate new skin growth, such as comfrey root extract; certain seaweeds and agents to help microcirculation, including arnica and rosemary. These herbs can be found ready made up in products from a good health shop or you can obtain a herbalist's prescription. They are far more effective external preparations than anything available within conventional medicine, which treats bedsores with zinc oxide and barrier creams. The herbal preparations can always be rubbed in before the barrier creams.

Sleeplessness

Sleeplessness denies the body the best time for healing, since sleep is a time when the body switches from doing things to mending and house-cleaning. If sleeplessness is due to noise and disturbance bring earplugs or better, a personal cassette recorder with relaxation tapes. Refuse sedatives. They have side effects, they impose an extra stress on the liver, steal nutrients, prevent self-care and inhibit recovery. Breathing exercises and relaxation in hospital (see page 72) are the best methods. One variation of yoga breathing that is especially helpful in inducing sleep is to breathe slowly into the stomach. Concentrate on the rise and fall of the stomach and the natural flow of breath into the stomach and out of it. If sleep still eludes you it is important not to worry. It is often a temporary natural response to disturbances, upset rhythms, or a lack of fresh air and exercise.

If you would like a mild herbal calmative, try strong chamomile tea before you go to bed. In one study patients were given a strong chamomile tea before heart catheterization. Several actually fell asleep during what is usually an uncomfortable procedure. If chamomile tea does not work there is still something stronger and yet much safer than sedatives – this is valerian root. In contrast to chamomile tea it cannot usually be bought in tea bags although you may find it as part of night-time herbal mixtures. Your companion can always bring a flask in the evening. Incidentally, try not to have stimulating coffee, tea, or Coca-Cola within four hours of bedtime. Herb teas are a much healthier replacement.

Indigestion, heartburn and gas

These conditions occur because of drugs, anaesthetics, change of diet, stomach infections and tension. Antacids do not work very well, stop absorption of valuable nutrients and can worsen digestion. Instead take slippery elm, marshmallow root, or Irish moss. They are soothing and at the same time promote healing in all the tissues. Peppermint tea relieves cramp and nausea and peppermint oil even relieves irritable bowel syndrome. Bitter herbs such as gentian and wormwood stimulate the appetite and improve digestion.

For gas you can use charcoal tablets, an old-time remedy that works. But aromatic spices, particularly cinnamon, ginger, aniseed and fennel seed are a very good way of relieving gas and settling the stomach, particularly because they are warming, benefiting the circulation, and also anti-infective in case of stomach infection. They help absorption of food and medicines. You can add these aromatics to any hot drink at one third to one quarter teaspoonful a time. Ginger is also effective at treating nausea. We discuss this in the next chapter.

Constipation

A common hospital problem. It can be dealt with partly by a diet with a great deal of roughage of different kinds, especially vegetables, salads and fresh fruit. Instead of conventional laxatives use linseed tea, a teaspoonful of isphaghula husk (plantago seed) or commercial laxative herb mixtures.

Headaches

Headaches arise from constipation, from toxins in the blood that haven't cleared, from stuffy atmosphere and positively charged air ions, from tension and stress and a variety of other causes. You should refuse strong cheeses or cocoa if you have recurrent headaches in hospital and use tiger balm, or oils of mint, eucalyptus, cajuput or rosemary, rubbing them into the temples, and massaging the nape of the neck. Herb teas or tablets consisting of dandelion, echinacea and St Johns Wort (Hypericum) are effective blood purifiers and can relieve headaches resulting from accumulated waste products in the blood. Juniper and parsley seed are natural ways of washing out these toxins from the blood. Headache symptoms are mostly the direct result of inflammatory processes in blood vessels in the head, and can be partly allayed by the deep relaxation we described above, by quiet and dark.

Tiredness and debility

Much tiredness and debility is the result of specific insults to health in hospital – poor digestion and absorption, poor diet, toxins and drug side effects, stress or shock to the system as in surgery and so on. Some of this tiredness is natural and leads to recovering sleep. The primary task is to remove the causes of fatigue by good diet, (page 76), supplements (page 81), yoga (page 69), or acupuncture (page 116).

When you are on the road to recovery extra vitality is certainly most helpful and it can be provided by Oriental restorative herbs. The most famous is ginseng, which has been well tried for this purpose. Ginseng used to be more of a myth than a medicine; now it is a mixture of the two. It is one of the best preventive and restorative remedies known. It is used to increase energy and alertness during chronic illness, recovery, weakness and old age. It is known to act on the hormonal circuitry of the body to prevent the harmful effects of stress, and to adjust the physiology – including blood sugar, blood pressure, the metabolism and body temperature. Its use against exhaustion has been supported by a great many scientific studies and applied in practice. In Soviet hospitals and in the Far East, ginseng or its relatives are used to give strength to recovering patients and prevent complications. In one study of 120 patients in a hospital in Seoul, Korea, who underwent serious abdominal or gynaecological surgery, half were given the active ingredients of ginseng and half a placebo. Those treated with ginseng had better liver function, put on weight faster and felt better. Similar studies have been carried out in Russia with a related herb, eleutherococcus.

Ginseng, or the Russian herb eleutherococcus, are ideal recovery herbs and should be in the tray of remedies your nurse brings round. It would save a lot of NHS money. However since you have to buy ginseng, and it is expensive, here are some rules. Buy whole roots or root pieces; if not available buy thick paste extract or ground root. Never buy instant tea. Choose Asian rather than

European brands. Asian red ginseng is better than white and well worth the extra money, but it must be a Korean or Chinese product. You should start taking ginseng in the recovery phase and *not* when you have a fever or infection. A dose of one gram a day is minimum. Eleutherococcus is cheaper and though it is effective as a restorative in bringing back vital functions, it is not so stimulating, so you may not notice the result as quickly as with ginseng. There is another reason to take these herbs which we describe below.

How to protect your immunity and prevent infections in hospital

Hospitals are pretty dangerous places to be ill. The Centre for Health Economics at the University of York, in the UK, recently confirmed that one in ten patients in hospital receive an infection there that they didn't have before, costing the NHS some £115 million per year. In the US some authorities say that it could be more than one in ten. Professor Schimpff, of the University of Maryland School of Medicine, suggested that 137,500 people die from pneumonia caught in US hospitals every year. In fact these hospital-born infections (HBI) led to the discovery of the existence of germs in the first place.

The fact is that all kinds of diseased fluids, fecal matter, discarded tissues, rubbish, food, diapers, catheters and so on are collected by people who go in and out of wards; that beds, stethoscopes, hospital equipment, lavatories and washbasins are in intimate contact with patient after patient, and that air conditioning and heating stir up and blow in dust and germs all over the place.

Recent hospital outbreaks of Legionnaires Disease, a very unusual and fatal infection, were traced to the alien germs hiding in the air conditioning systems. The hospital is the breeding ground of completely new and antibiotic-resistant organisms mostly because of indiscriminate use of antibiotics. The most worrisome is a new strain of the common-or-garden staphylococcus called MSRA, dubbed by the media as super-staph, which is resistant to virtually all the available antibiotics. It has been identified in 132 hospitals all over

England and has led to wards and Intensive Care Units being closed. It is rife in US hospitals too, and in the US the worst fears of doctors has happened – the creation of new strains of bacteria that are resistant to all known antibiotics. At present these bacteria are uncommon, but if they spread, we may be back to a medieval situation where patients die in hospital because of a cut finger.

It is also true that patients in hospital are often so weak and vulnerable that they catch infections even from the germs that normally live on the outside of their body as harmlessly as ants in the grass. Medical specialists, of course, cite this as the main reason for the high rate of infections. But it is not at all as good an excuse as it sounds. For a good deal of the weakness and vulnerability comes from the hospital milieu itself. After all, you don't need to worry about getting pneumonia along with treatment by an acupuncturist or homoeopath.

It is not that hospital doctors want to lower resistance, they simply don't understand how to raise it. The philosophy and practice of modern medicine, as it is taught in medical schools, is to look for specific causes of disease and attack them rather than look for a weakness or vulnerability to disease and prevent it.

So you will have to look after your own resistance, to help the natural doctor already within you or as Hippocrates described it: the *Vix Medicatrix Naturae* (natural healing force). The body machinery that shields you from infections is called the immune system. It is a flexible defensive system, capable of reacting to all kinds of alien agents which threaten the body, from viruses to bacteria, from smoke particles in smokers' lungs to the mutated cancer cells that may crop up in their bodies. It consists, broadly, of protective proteins which circulate in the blood, and different kinds of white cells which are made in the thymus gland and spleen and distributed everywhere, especially in the lymph.

We have already described how the immune system is weakened by negative mental states including fear, tension, overwork, anxiety, and exhaustion, all summed up by the catchword 'stress'. Stress is one cause of the vulnerability of hospital patients and we have described the importance of reducing stress in hospital and methods of achieving this. Poor nutrition is another factor, and it is known that undernourished patients in hospital are more likely to acquire infections there. We have described the importance of vitamin C, A, zinc, and B vitamins as well as a good general nutrition, in enabling the immunity to fight effectively.

A further cause of immune deterioration is drugs. No one really knows which drugs affect your resistance, because lingering side effects such as chronic infections and a feeling of being run-down are not taken very seriously in conventional medicine and not properly monitored. However white blood cells are known to be reduced as a result of antifungal antibiotics such as erythromycin; tricyclic antidepressants; certain nonsteroid anti-inflammatory drugs such as indomethacin; any preparation containing cortico-steroids; and phenothiazine tranquilizers. Any chemotherapeutic agent will have drastic effects on immunity.

Although it would be unwise to be vexed and paranoid, seeing a lethal bug behind every curtain, there are a few simple pre-cautions that you can take to reduce your vulnerability to germs:

- Fresh circulating air is important. Try to have as much as possible by opening windows. Remember air ions.
- Don't travel around too much. You don't know what you will be picking up in the nooks and crannies, and bringing back to bed with you.
- Try to minimize physical contact with other patients.
- Take showers rather than baths and maintain personal hygiene.
- Try not to take broad spectrum antibiotics needlessly. If you have a mild fever, don't automatically suppress it with aspirin and assume it is a dangerous infection. It may be the body cleaning and defending itself naturally. Ask the doctor to do a lab test to identify the bug before giving you antibiotics. Tell him that if it is a minor problem you would prefer to get over it by yourself.

Besides the self-care methods described above, the real power to aid your immunity exists in the plant kingdom. Here there are a wide range of active medicinal agents for this purpose, which your doctor will know nothing about. Because of the variety of medicines and because restoring immunity is more complex than, say, treating constipation, you would be well advised to seek a consultation with a herbalist or naturopath. Here follow some remedies that you can take to strengthen immunity, besides garlic which we have already mentioned. It would be best if you could select and take the correct herbs to fit your specific needs. However in the absence of personal advice from an alternative practitioner, you could try ready made formulations that contain any of the plants described below as their chief constituent.

Mistletoe

Viscum album or mistletoe is a classic plant medicine of Northern Europe, made famous as the holy Druid plant, growing like a transplant on the oak. It is used as a traditional anti-cancer remedy working by encouraging the immunity. A team of scientists at the Department of Immunology of the University of Utrecht found that it increases the weight of the organs associated with immunity, the thymus and spleen, and rapidly accelerates the production of antibodies. Mistletoe can be given as a shot in the arm to the immunity, although it is strong, and should be under the advice of a herbalist. The usual daily dose is three grams of powdered leaves or 0.5 millilitres of a tincture.

Propolis

Propolis is not a herb but an anti-infective material which bees collect from the sap of certain trees. They plaster it over the hive where it helps to cleanse the hive and protect young bees from disease. Plant-derived substances in propolis called flavonoids are capable of directly stimulating the immune system to make antibodies. Propolis is harmless. It can be taken every day as a nugget held in the mouth next to the gum until it eventually dissolves. It is available as tablets.

Echinacae, Golden Seal, Sarsparilla and Pau d'arco

Herbs used in Western herbalism to promote immunity come under the category of 'alteratives' or 'blood purifiers', lumping together the attacking of an infection with the removal of its products. Four immune stimulating plants for internal housekeeping are: Echinacae (*Echinacea angustifolium*), Golden Seal (*Hydrastis canadensis*), Sarsparilla (*Smilax*), and Pau d'arco. These should be taken as powders in capsules, 1 gm three times a day. Perhaps the best of them is echinacea which is now available as freeze dried flower and root extract, with guaranteed potency. There are other mild Western herbs which you can take to nourish the tissues that build immunity. They are gentle and suitable for self-treatment but may not be sufficient by themselves. Examples include dandelion and angelica.

While the West has 100 years of developing drugs that cure diseases, China has several thousand years experience of developing drugs that prevent them. While the West values its most powerful agents such as cortisone, the East values mild, safe remedies such as liquorice, calling them kingly remedies. The unbroken development of Chinese medicine has allowed unparalleled sophistication. They now know hundreds of plants, each of which can activate, depress, divert, concentrate, disperse or alter any one of a large number of different physiological processes in the body. The immunity, being one of the most critical to health, is of particular interest to Chinese practitioners and they have discovered many plants that affect it in different ways. We discuss the plants that restore immunity destroyed by chemotherapy and radiotherapy in Chapter 5. Here are some Chinese 'tonic' plants that can be used to strengthen and bolster immunity while you are at risk from less drastic medical circumstances such as a stay in hospital after surgery.

Eleutherococcus

The immune-protective and immune-stimulating properties of eleutherococcus has long been suspected by Soviet scientists, based on their laboratory tests. This led to an enormous trial in which it was given to 14,000 workers at the Volzhsky car factory in Togliatti. There was a dramatic reduction in the usual infections. Its action has been described as 'adaptogenic' that is, helping the body to regulate itself and to deal with stress; it is particularly useful where stress is seen as the cause of weak resistance. Take eleutherococcus in preference to ginseng where you wish to support the immunity and resistance, without stimulation or arousal.

Angelica sinensis (Tang Kwei)
Often described as the 'female ginseng', it is recommended for restoring energy and vitality, but in females rather than males, for whom regular ginseng is better. It has been found to have strong immune protective effects, by activating different kinds of white cells and antibody-forming spleen cells, and is used in China for this purpose.

Liquorice
Liquorice can be very effective, surprisingly, at promoting antibody production and the regulation of white cells. However, it can also, under certain conditions, depress the immunity, so it should only be taken for immune defence in a professionally prepared herb mixture. It is an excellent general tonic after illness.

Panax ginseng
This is true ginseng, the best recovery medicine there is, particularly in cases of severe debility, poor immune function, and weakness from disease. It increases the number of white cells in the blood, increases their general responsiveness, and helps spleen and liver provide energy for immunological reactions. Ginseng is rather stimulating, and in some cases, as in young men with plenty of energy, or in those of a 'hot' agitated disposition, it would be better to take a non-stimulating immune restorative. In such cases you can take eleutherococcus. Another possibility is American ginseng (*Panax quinquefolium*) which is a non-stimulating general tonic. Its effects on immunity have not been scientifically investigated, but judging from traditional sources and the nature of the plant constituents I suspect it has a some of the immune-restoring qualities of Panax ginseng.

Tang-Shen, Ganoderma, Reishi,
An Oriental plant that is used as a substitute for ginseng and is of considerable benefit to the immunity is *Codonopsis lanceolate*, or Tang-Shen. It is not stimulating but nourishes the immunity. Ganoderma and Reishi mushrooms contain some very important immune-stimulating compounds, and are now becoming available in the West. Studies in China and the USSR suggest that

Ganoderma mushroom the Oriental 'Mushroom of Immortality' may be one of the most effective general immune supporters known. There are a number of less well known Oriental remedies which are potentially very effective. However they are hard to obtain in the West, and can only be obtained with the help of a practitioner of Oriental medicine.

In general, you will be able to find the above Oriental herbs in your local health shop. They should be taken at a dose of 1 gm two or three times a day. You can also obtain commercial mixtures which combine alternative Chinese tonic herbs so that the total is much better than the sum of its parts. For example ginseng may provide energy, but when combined with ginger it aids the circulation so that the effects of ginseng are spread properly, while added liquorice regulates water balance, to harmonize the other two. Chinese companies export some mixtures, such as Shou wu Chih (a source of angelica) or Peking Royal Jelly Liquid (a source of Codonopsis together with Royal Jelly, a useful tonic in its own right) or Shih Chuan Ta Pu Tonic pills (a mixture of the best Oriental herbs for immune support).

Chapter Four

SURGERY

At knifepoint

'I'm sure it's nothing, but just to be on the safe side we'll have it out.' There is something alarming about these comforting words addressed to us by a complete stranger in a white coat.

Surgery is the best of modern medicine: the highly skilled professionals, the elaborate technical backup, the detailed, con-centrated knowledge of the offending anatomy, the wizardry of repairing damaged tissues, and the computerised monitoring equipment. If the hospital is the temple of medicine, the operating theatre is its altar.

Yet by the same token it is the worst of medicine: the highly skilled professionals have no real contact with you and little under-standing of the real causes of illness. The machinery causes stress. The concentration on an anatomical piece means that you your-self are merely a sort of carrier of your problem – 'the prostate in bed 7'. Management is at the expense of communication, computers at the expense of touching, medication prevents prevention.

Surgery is often a vital life-saving procedure. There would be little argument about the 20 per cent of surgery that is emergency work. An emergency is an emergency. But if your surgery belongs to the other 80 per cent you will be faced by a difficult decision about an irreversible procedure, (you can't put back whatever is removed) which carries risks and discomforts.

The first question to ask: is it really necessary? This may seem a strange question: surely doctors wouldn't be recommending it if it wasn't necessary would they? Unfortunately they do. Surgeons know how to do surgery, and if you go to one with a health problem, surgery is likely to be his recommendation. Ignorance of alternative, psychosomatic or preventive healing methods leads to a great deal of unnecessary surgery, as surgeon Bernie Segal has pointed out in his books. And if the surgeon has the added incentive of being paid for each surgery performed, the number of operations goes up three times. A US Senate Committee set up to investigate unnecessary operations reported that 2.4 million unnecessary operations were performed in America each year at a cost of four billion dollars. Other experts put the figure at six million unnecessary operations. Just the existence of a watchdog hospital committee to check whether surgery is necessary or not has been found to reduce surgery by two thirds.

In the UK, under the National Health Service, paying surgeons for each operation would be as unthinkable as paying policemen for each arrest. There is therefore half the amount of surgery than in the US. Even so, 20,000 useless appendix removals are performed each year. Tonsil removal was very popular some years ago, until it was realised that children without tonsils suffer as much infection if not more than those with them, and they have a four times greater risk of a cancer called Hodgkin's disease. It turns out that tonsils are inflamed only because they are doing their job of filtering out smoke and pollution (they are more swollen in children of parents who smoke). Still, 90,000 tonsils are removed in the UK every year, and in many of these cases a simple change of diet or a clean environment would have solved the problem. There are also new fashions which have not been scientifically examined to see if they are really necessary. A new one is tympanostomy – the puncture of the ear drum and drainage of the ear channel for persistent ear infections in children. Again, a change of diet can often provide a permanent cure.

Clearly, if at your first meeting with a specialist he recommends surgery, it is doubly necessary to follow the guidelines suggested in the previous chapter about how to check his recommendation. That is, to take time off in order to understand the problem and the treatment fully. The specialist should tell you if you run any risks by delaying the treatment. In any event, in the UK you will have a long wait for non-emergency surgery, which no doubt saves a great many unnecessary operations. During your waiting period, learn from friends, past patients, books, health magazines, self-help groups, patients and practitioners of alternative medicine, about the alternative treatment options, the particular type of surgery recommended (success rate, types of side effects, recovery time, etc.), the record of the recommended hospital and surgeon.

You need to ask yourself:

- Whether the diagnosis you have been given really seems to fit your situation.
- What are the existing options for treatment?
- What are the chances of success with each treatment, and what are the side effects?
- Why the disease may have appeared in you at this time.
- Whether it is part of a pattern of recurring disease in your life.
- Whether there are suitable alternative non-conventional treatment methods.

It is of interest to list the most over-used operations. These are given in the table below. My comments are all based on published medical research.

The most common unnecessary operations

Operation	Reasons for doubt
Appendix removal	Three quarters of all appendices removed in Germany found normal.
Back operations	Surgery often has no advantage over safer treatments e.g. physiotherapy. *Lancet* says 60 per cent of operations unnecessary
Biopsy	If for cancer, may spread it. Can sometimes be done by your GP.
Breast removal	Removal of whole breast does not increase survival over removal of lump only, or quarter of breast. Review of 8000 cases show no differences in survival between any of the procedures. Stress of surgery can spread the cancer. Surgeons now confused and patients turning to alternatives.

	Breast removal traumatic: quarter of all patients suicidally depressed.
Heart by-pass	Recovery slow. Scarring and depression common. Patients do not live longer after operation unless blockage severe. European Coronary Surgery Study Group showed benefits marginal if at all, *The Journal of the American Medical Association* states that 50 per cent are unnecessary.
Circumcision	*British Medical Journal* says it's safer at home than in hospital.
Gallstone removal	One in 30 elderly die from operation. Leaves scars and pain. But 'quiet' stones often removed unnecessarily. New safe ultrasonic method available.
Heart/kidney transplants	Russian roulette. Alternative methods at early stages can also save hearts and kidneys.
Hernia	Four times more dangerous to have operation than to go without.
Hysterectomy	Only one in five clinically fully justified in US where half a million are performed every year. 30 per cent of cases infected, 40 per cent depressed.
Tonsils/adenoids removal	Not necessary except where danger of blockage.
Tympanostomy (ear drum punction and drainage)	An unnecessary fashion, like tonsil removal. Blockages treatable by diet.

If you agree to surgery there are a number of questions you should ask about it, in addition to those discussed in the previous chapter. These questions are directed towards finding out more about the procedure, and if the surgeon is the right man for the job. In addition it gives you some indication of the seriousness of the operation. The more serious the operation, the longer it takes, and the longer it will take to recover afterwards.

There are sometimes new procedures which you should go for if they are safer and gentler. For example it is worth looking around for a centre that can remove gallstones safely in an ultrasonic bath rather than take an offer of an early surgery. A new procedure called resectoscopy has now been approved by the FDA to remove fibroids in the womb. It is far better than a hysterectomy.

You should ask:

1   How long will the actual operation take?
2   What is the complication rate for this procedure?
3   How many of these operations have you done? (If under ten don't use this surgeon/consultant.)
4   How long will it take me to recover, and how long to be back at work?
5   What should I do after the operation to promote recovery?
6   Will you do the surgery yourself or will you just supervise?
7   Will you be able to recommend a second opinion (see previous chapter)?

Many operations that used to require a stay in hospital can now be carried out on an outpatient basis. This is partly from pressure to reduce expenditure, and because of more advanced techniques. Procedures such as biopsy, hernia repair, varicose vein removal, cytoscopy, arthoscopy, and many others can be done without the risks, expense, and stress of a hospital stay. If you have the choice, it is usually better to have the procedure done as an outpatient. But make sure that full hospital facilities are available nearby in case of emergencies.

Don't forget that surgery always carries risks, even if slight, and the surgeon is required by law to inform you about them. Also, you will be required, before surgery, to sign a form stating that you are giving your informed consent. Obviously, if you are not receiving full answers to your questions you should remind the consultant that you cannot give informed consent unless you are informed.

In this crucial period in which you are making your decisions, keep an open mind. It would be wise to follow the advice of Dr Robert Mendelsohn, given in his book *MalePractice*:

■ Don't assume that the operation is necessary.
■ Don't be deceived by a well-polished air of confidence.
■ Don't assume that all the treatment choices have been considered.
■ Don't assume that the surgery will actually make you feel better.
■ Don't assume that the surgeon cannot make mistakes.

Preparation for surgery

Once you have decided to have a certain operation performed by a certain surgeon you can leave the doubts behind. You have made your decision and you can, and should, trust both your body and the surgeon to do their best. Encourage the doctors, and share with them the burden of getting you well.

It is important to come to an operation as fit as possible. This will help to eliminate the anaesthetics quickly after the surgery and hasten healing. You will need plenty of exercise. Cut out alcohol, unnecessary drugs and junk foods for a month before-hand to improve the condition of your liver. Try to reduce coffee and tea intake. It is known that people who consume a lot of caffeine recover more slowly from anaesthetics. It is commonly assumed that the time to take a holiday is after the operation. In fact it is equally important to take a holiday before, so as to arrive well rested and well prepared. Your nutrition should be top class, concentrating on proteins and vitamins. For presurgery nutritional supplementation, for two weeks prior to surgery, take at least 2 gm vitamin C per day (with bioflavonoids), vitamin E, B complex and minerals especially magnesium and zinc.

Remember to prepare your psychological as well as physical health by learning relaxation or arranging for hypnosis as described below.

In addition, you should prepare your surgeon by letting him know your special requirements. As described in the previous chapter, you should inform him of the supplements and herbs you are going to be taking, request any special skills such as hypnosis or massage which you wish to find among the medical staff, and inform him of your natural mindedness and intention to minimize drugs.

If you are going to be on an intravenous drip for more than a few hours, and cannot take oral vitamin supplements, request beforehand that the surgeon arrange for vitamin C, B complex and minerals to be added to your drip. It is possible but not routine.

Consider the timing of the operation carefully. It should be at a time when you will have a supportive companion available and at a time when you feel at your best mentally, physically and even astrologically! Women should have surgery during the middle of the menstrual cycle (days 7 to 20) when the immunity is highest, and never, if possible, during menstruation, when you are at your lowest ebb.

Rights and consent

Despite any pressure put on you, no one can force you to sign anything, to do anything or to receive any treatment. If you are not getting the procedure agreed on previously, you can refuse it. However the hospital can also refuse to treat you – *you do not have a right to a particular treatment, you only have a right to competent treatment.* Under the NHS you have no right to a particular surgeon, but you do of course if you have paid for him. You do not lose your rights by signing consent forms or other forms.

A general consent form may be handed to you on admission. You should sign this form, as otherwise you may not be admitted. However you should add statements or strike out those which you do not wish to sign, especially any that appear to reduce the liability of the hospital in case things go wrong. If the admissions staff object, call the hospital administrator and explain your case. A specific consent form will also be presented to you before the operation in addition to any general consent to treatment you may have signed on admission to the hospital. The consent form is often, through carelessness, given just before the operation when you are too nervous or drugged to know how to handle it. Therefore ask your doctor or intern for it beforehand.

■ The consent form must describe exactly the procedure you agreed upon beforehand with your surgeon.
■ It could have a blanket clause of this type:
   'I also consent to such further or alternative operative measures as may be found to be necessary during the course of the operation, and to the administration of a general, or other anaesthetic for any of these purposes.'
   As a wise patient, wary of unnecessary surgery, you may want to strike this out. You are free to do so.

- You may choose to strike out the clause (in teaching hospitals) permitting observers and spectators.
- You may strike out the clause permitting disposal of material removed during the operation, for example if you want a second opinion on a biopsy sample.
- Do not sign that you have been fully informed unless that is the case.
- You may wish to add a sentence that you consent only if the surgeon whom you expect to do the operation will actually do it.

What is going to happen?

If your operation is scheduled in the morning, you will have arrived in hospital at least the day before. In the evening the anaesthetist will normally drop in to see you in your ward for a brief chat. He is responsible for your well-being during the operation; the surgeon is only concerned with the surgery itself. Therefore the anaesthetist will wish to get to know your physical and mental fitness, for a general anaesthetic is quite a shock to the system. The heart needs to be healthy to keep up a good circulation while under anaesthesia, the liver and metabolism need to break down and remove the anaesthetic. The anaesthetist will therefore check if you have had a heart attack, circulatory problems, diabetes, hepatitis or other liver problems or allergies. You may be asked if you prefer a local anaesthetic if it is an option for that particular operation. He will check how anxious you are. Almost everyone is nervous, and research has shown that one out of two people are afraid of dying on the operating table. A good anaesthetist may indirectly determine your mood and will postpone the operation if you are really pessimistic about your chances.

The next day, an hour before the operation, you would normally be given tranquilizers. Then you will be wheeled into a waiting room and shortly before the operation you will be given the 'premed' – drugs such as tubocurarine and atropine to relax the muscles to prevent muscle spasms, and dry up secretions. If you have agreed to have a local anaesthetic this will now be done through an injection into the muscles. If it is a nerve block (epidural) it will be an injection into the space around the spinal cord. This can be a little painful for a brief moment, after which it is painless.

For a general anaesthetic, an injection of a barbiturate such as thiopental is given to put you to sleep, and then a gaseous anaesthetic continues throughout the operation. This is usually nitrous oxide/ oxygen, and halothane. The state of anaesthesia is somewhere between sleep and a coma. It is dreamless and on waking you will feel that no time has passed.

The anaesthetic is timed to run out just after the operation. You are taken into a recovery room or Intensive Care Unit, and the sister may call your name to wake you up.

Realistic expectations

It is advisable to know the real risks of surgery, just to avoid fearing the unreal ones. Around one in 100 people do not pull through surgery, mostly those who are old or very sick anyway. Post surgical infection is the main complication, affecting up to 30 per cent of patients in certain operations such as hysterectomies. There is a small risk of errors or viral diseases arising from blood transfusions. A major problem in surgery is internal bleeding. Shock, blood clots that wander or slips-of-the-knife are other, unusual, physical risks. A long-term risk of surgery is scarring, which may cause postoperative pain, discomfort and ill-health. It is often unrecognized by the medical profession.

Modern anaesthesia is very safe. Yet as with all medical procedures there can be risks and discomforts which you should know about. Anaesthesia is a procedure that can often have unpleasant immediate side effects after you awake, which soon go away. These include vomiting, nausea, trembling and shaking, dizziness, disorientation. There are ways to reduce these effects which are described below. However you should know that these after effects of anaesthetics are common and completely normal, and you need not be disturbed by the anxiety that something may be going wrong.

Possible side effects of anaesthesia are proportional to the length of the operation. Psychological complications are the most common and often least recognised risk of anaesthesia. For example, minor brain damage can be quite common in cardiac surgery, arising from toxic residues of anaesthetics, sterilizing gases or plastic tubes, and clots or bubbles in the circulation. There can be confusion, weakness or long bouts of depression, which are often considered more or less normal. In any case mental function may take weeks to get back to normal. This shows especially in the ability to solve problems, in memory, and language skills. A crossword enthusiast may find himself inexplicably stumped for two months. The mental slowness is very clear to any health worker up to four days after an operation. With special tests a psychologist can distinguish those who have had a general anaesthetic for six weeks afterwards.

Occasionally you may notice a physical problem soon after the operation, for example numbness in a limb, a strained muscle in the neck, legs or arms, or even a dislocation. These may arise from the anaesthetist failing to position you properly on the table, resulting in a trapped nerve or twisted limb. Very often a physiotherapist can help you to regain mobility. Massage and osteopathy can be very useful in such cases.

One example of this can be seen in the experience of Mary, who went into hospital shortly after her 42nd birthday to have a hysterectomy because of uterine polyps:

'I discovered that something was dreadfully wrong about a day after when I tried to raise my hand to push hair off my face, and found that it flopped back, ragdoll fashion, from less than shoulder height. I told the nurse who couldn't have been less interested. When I tried to lever myself to a sitting position the left arm collapsed under me. I don't mind admitting I was terrified and started trying to find out what I could do about it. Having got no sense out of the nurse I showed my gynecologist what was happening, and he arranged that a neurologist should see me.

The neurologist, Dr Henry, admitted that possibly a nerve had been trapped during the anaesthetic and that an orthopaedic surgeon might be able to help. I just couldn't bear to see another surgeon, so when I left hospital I saw an osteopath. He said it was certainly a trapped nerve.

After three sessions of treatment at weekly intervals I had full mobility and sensation, the thumb being the last part to return to normal feeling. I now play the piano and lute, go riding, swim twice a week, and lead a full and active life.'

Your talk with the anaesthesiologist/anaesthetist

The anaesthesiologist is a physician who is trained in the giving of anaesthetics and in supervising the patient's general condition during the operation. An anaesthetist is a specially trained nurse or other medical staff and is junior to the anaesthesiologist. If you have a choice, have a long operation, or have paid for him, make sure that the anaesthesiologist himself will be supervising you, and not leaving it to the anaesthetist.

It is essential that you ask the anaesthesiologist/anaesthetist to give you more time than the perfunctory five minutes. State that you are the kind of patient who will benefit from full prior information and that you request it. These are the issues to bring up:

- Ask for a full description of the procedure.
- Ask if it is possible to use a local anaesthetic instead. If so request it.
- What are the tablets, premedication, and anaesthetics?
- How long will you be 'out'?
- What are possible long term physical/psychological side effects?
- Make sure that you relate all your significant health problems especially any heart and circulatory problems, liver problems, or past liver diseases, alcohol or drug consumption, asthma, diabetes, or allergies. These conditions increase the risk of an anaesthetic. For example if someone has had a heart attack within six months prior to anaesthesia, there is a one in 20 chance of having another one during or just after the anaesthetic. In such cases discuss the risks with the anaesthesiologist/anaesthetist. If necessary consider again alternative medicine instead of surgery, or plan for acupuncture anaesthesia (see below, page 115).

Tell the anaesthesiologist/anaesthetist about your intention to use pre-anaesthetic relaxation skills or other stress reduction methods (see below) instead of tranquilizers. Remember that tranquilizers make it impossible to prepare yourself and relax. You lose all clarity. They do not necessarily calm you down. You might feel extremely anxious but cannot show it and cannot express it. The anxiety is frozen. In addition they have side effects of their own. Many patients feel knocked out and need to recover more from tranquilizers after-effects than from the anaesthetic. Tranquilizers should be taken only in extreme cases of panic when no help such as hypnosis is available.

Ask for as much quiet as possible and for encouraging things to be said to you when you are under the anaesthetic. Failing that ask for cotton wool to put in your ears. You may not remember what went on in the operating theatre, but some part of you does register comments, especially where it concerns your fate. These can act as unconscious suggestions to affect your recovery. Eve, a physiotherapist of my acquaintance, gave an anaesthetist a short poem about sleep to read to her as she went under. At first he was embarrassed to intone pastoral phrases about snoozing on a summer afternoon but now he uses the poem with everyone.

How to deal with stress and anxiety before operations

Surgery is the most stressful of all hospital experiences. You are in unfamiliar surroundings, without control over yourself, with your very life and integrity in the hands of strangers whose competence you can only guess at. You could be frightened of the possibility of pain, damage or even death, and there is usually no one to hold your hand through the experience. The anticipation of surgery is known to release a flood of stress hormones which reduce resistance. The longer patients wait in hospital for an operation the weaker they can therefore become. There has been a great deal of research showing that the more anxious a patient is, the more difficult is the operation; there is extra pain and longer recovery and recuperation.

As hospital doctors know little about stress or anxiety and its consequences, they can only prescribe tranquilizers. In this way, staff escape from the need to give psychological preparation for surgery. You have to help yourself. A great deal depends on your advance preparation for surgery, and the frame of mind you bring to the hospital. Those who are calm, confident and energetic, can often sail through the experience without batting an eyelid.

Such confidence can come partly from making sure you have done everything possible to select the treatment, and then feeling able to hand the rest over to the doctors. This confidence may seem like a will o'the wisp if you are sick, depressed and worried. However there are tricks to elicit it. Humour is a classical method. So is action. One man I knew was agonizing for ages over whether or not to have a heart by-pass operation. Careful preparation of the kind we have discussed gave him the answer that he should have it, as he didn't want to go through life 'waiting for the other shoe to drop'. His wife, a psychologist, told him to write everything down, both before the operation and afterwards; what he felt, what he saw, what were his values, his reactions. This made him involved and important, and built up his confidence.

One of the best ways of preparing yourself is relaxation training, which should be initiated some weeks before the surgery. Research has clearly shown that relaxation is more effective than tranquilizers in preventing stress and anxiety before surgery. However in some cases the anxiety is too strong to allow proper relaxation. Another method can achieve the same results as deep relaxation even when you are in a state of strong anxiety or fear. This is hypnosis. It has the advantage that it is done to you, rather than a training that you must prepare for yourself.

Hypnosis before and after surgery

Very often a person who has surgery is in a crisis – an emotional, energetic or personal crisis. The crisis takes away the will to help yourself. It could lead to a difficult operation and a slow recovery. Hypnosis can cut through the panic and open the gate to inner resources. Doctors use it mostly for pain relief, relaxation, for psychosomatic disease such as migraine and in reducing anxiety. It is very valuable with children before surgery or dentistry, both because they are such good subjects and because they are much more vulnerable to the fear, shock and pain produced by medical treatment.

Hypnosis, like relaxation training, has been shown to lead to more successful surgery with less pain. Anaesthetists report that hypnotized patients need less anaesthetic and less narcotics after the operation. Hypnosis can be seen as a powerful way of marshaling your unconscious self-healing abilities. It helps you get back in touch with yourself and introduces a positive and confident frame of mind. Hypnosis before operations is no longer the rarity it once was. Indeed there are certain hospitals, especially in the US, where hypnosis is used as a matter of course. One such is the University of California Medical School at Sacramento.

Hypnosis is a method of bypassing the thinking, worrying mind and reaching down to deeper layers. Often this is quite simply done by suggesting relaxation using pictures, numbers or repetitive sounds or images. Hypnotists can even induce a relaxed hypnotic state while talking about the weather. You could be taken on a brief journey into childhood memories. As one elderly lady said, who was doing rather poorly after cardiac surgery, 'What was most useful was talking about being up the valleys. I told him about where I was born.'

Hypnosis goes beyond relaxation by implanting specific suggestions in the unconscious mind: suggestions that you will feel less pain and recover more quickly with less side effects; that the whole operation will be a quick and easy event and that you will soon be on your feet feeling very bright. During the hypnosis you will feel relaxed and detached. The hypnotist will suggest that you feel like that when you go into the operation and as you come out of it. One hypnotist I know visited his friend who had been in an accident and was carried unconscious into the theatre. He awoke from the anaesthetic shouting and fearful, tearing the stitches. The hypnotist hypnotized his friend (who did not recognise him) by talking about rest, warmth and comfort. The friend slept immediately. Later he implanted suggestions of a speedy recovery, and this occurred.

People vary in their suggestibility. Those who are suggestible will sometimes react dramatically to instructions given while in deep trance. Yet almost everyone can be helped by hypnosis – one orthopaedic surgeon said that hypnosis allowed 90 per cent of minor fractures to be set in a casualty department without any anaesthetic at all.

It would be best to undergo hypnosis once or twice before you enter hospital as it is important to build a rapport with the hypnotist. He can also teach you to do it yourself. Then, receive 15 to 20 minutes of hypnosis in the ward an hour or two before the operation. There are at least 1000 doctors trained in hypnosis in hospitals and the community in the UK, and several thousand in the US. Ask the anaesthesiologist/anaesthetist if he can recommend a medical hypnotist from the hospital itself. If not, ask whether you can bring your own. If there is serious opposition, a non medical hypnotist can visit you in the guise of 'friend' or 'counsellor' before surgery.

Holding your hand

I asked a number of patients, alternative practitioners and nurses what they felt would be the greatest single help before and just after an operation. Most said: a good friend. People think of visitors coming after it is all over. A true friend is needed even more before it begins. A companion can be a source of encouragement, sympathy, and tireless assistance. 'When she couldn't walk to the toilet, I was her spine, when she despaired, I was her hope, when she needed peace, I was her guardian,' was how a friend described her care for her mother in hospital.

Hospitals don't always get along with visitors. They ought to, because visitors can profoundly reduce anxiety and stress. Researchers in the US have demonstrated how visitors can promote recovery: 'Visitors have reassured the patient about her impending surgery. Visitors have been a distraction...a type of relaxation.' The reaction to a friendly face can be dramatic. This is how Penny Brohn described her rescue during a lumpectomy under local anaesthetic in her book *Gentle Giants*:

'My lump didn't want to part company with me and stubbornly refused to co-operate with the surgeon's efforts. I bled a lot, everybody swabbed. The frown lines around the eyes over the mask deepened, the pain grew worse and worse. More and more anaesthetic made no difference, not to the breast that is, although I was almost paralyzed down the left-hand side for hours afterwards. Nasty clinking, clanking noises. More pain, more difficult to cope with. Relax, breathe properly, relax. Then comfort; the theatre sister, sitting next to me, putting her arms around me, murmuring encouragement, barking and snapping at my tormentors. I love her.'

Someone close to you is especially needed in the Intensive Care Unit (ICU). The sensory deprivation, the drugs, the stress and the machines make many patients feel as if they are going mad there. The staff are now trained to be more human, and to talk to patients to ease the psychological strain. But a caring companion is especially needed to help you keep contact with the real world and give essential human support.

Breathing before and after surgery

Controlled breathing is one of the most effective ways of calming yet energising the body and the mind, and reducing pain. This is why it is universally taught to mothers to ease birth. It is a great pity that it is not also taught to surgical patients. After surgery it is especially useful to help expel the toxic gases of the anaesthetic, clear the mind, help recovery and encourage a good night's sleep. This is how yoga student Alex Barclay recently described his recovery from by-pass surgery at the Harefield Hospital:

'I awoke a few minutes later as a dulcet voice asked me to breathe deeply in and slowly out and to retain the breath when asked. I had the feeling I was back in my yoga class doing breathing exercises, but having been prewarned by the physiotherapist I knew I was in the Intensive Care Unit and now was the time to have a multitude of drain tubes removed…Two days later I was out of bed, in a chair practicing physiotherapy, or yoga, since that was what it was … I have not the slightest doubt that without it I would have taken far longer to recover, and perhaps succumbed to intense post-operative depression.'

Two small surveys of cancer patients who have been helped by yoga breathing have been carried out in Cambridge. Several cancer patients reported that yoga had helped them calmly prepare for surgery and recover from the anaesthetic afterwards. 'Alternate nostril breathing after injection in preparation for the theatre was so successful that I lost consciousness even before being removed from the ward…' noted one patient.

The basic instructions on controlled, steady breathing have been given in the previous chapter, page 72. They should be learnt beforehand from a yoga teacher. In the postoperative period it is especially important to take slow steady regular breaths, filling the abdomen with air, and breathing out for twice as long as breathing in. This is to oxygenate the blood, start the intestines moving and bring blood to the organs. Don't breathe too hard and fast otherwise you may get dizzy from hyperventilation. Instead let the breath 'breathe you'.

After surgery in the chest or abdomen, coughing and strong full slow breathing will help lung function and clear out unwanted fluids. Hold the place of the suture if necessary to prevent pain and stress at that place while you breathe deeply. Dr Alan Hymes, a heart surgeon at the University of Minnesota, always teaches his patients this kind of breathing after heart surgery to reduce pain, depression and complications.

Spiritual or psychic healing

Spiritual or psychic healing is the giving of therapeutic energy by a trained or gifted healer. It is not designed to treat any specific health problem. However it can give a big boost to your self-healing capacity and hasten recovery and repair after surgery. In fact in some situations where recovery is slow and a patient may be deteriorating, healing has been known to cause a dramatic turn-around. There is something very subtle involved in healing. Patients who have been healed often report being much more comfortable, and feeling as if their scattered physical, psychological and spiritual selves have been put back together. Healing usually requires the healer to apply a very concentrated form of touch, with the hands placed on or just above the patient. In a recent clinical study, healing was tested for its ability to relieve post-operative pain. Patients who had dental surgery reported reduced pain intensity from four hours afterwards, if they had received healing, compared to similar surgery without healing. In neither case did the patients actually know whether they had had healing or not.

One less obvious but important role of healing is to repair the damage of surgery on a subtle level so that it will not recur as pain or ill-health later on. This is how one healer put it:

'Surgery can be emotionally draining, especially if it is the removal of part of the body to which there is a strong emotional tie, such as hysterectomy or mastectomy. This can lead to chronic tiredness and depression. I "see" this damage of surgery as a hole in the aura. I simply darn the hole like darning an old sock. The energy drain is plugged and the patient recovers.'

Healing can accomplish something else – it can work on a suture to prevent scarring. A very great deal of post-surgical pain, which can last for years, is due to the scars and the tissue memory of the damage. Through healing, tensions are released, circulation improves and nerves are repaired more quickly. One healer described how:

'I stroke the scar area for 20 minutes, warming it, and some-times the surgery is relived, trauma comes out and the patient cries. The memory of it is no longer locked in the tissues, which relax, and scarring is reduced. This is especially important in high-tension muscles such as those of the lower back, or the neck.'

Anaesthesia by acupuncture

There *are* alternatives to anaesthesia, besides the medieval one of a bottle of brandy and some stout attendants. The newspaper pictures of stomach or heart surgery performed in China under acupuncture anaesthesia are perfectly true. The Chinese have now performed a million operations under acupuncture anaesthesia. The dramas of patients under acupuncture anaesthesia chatting to the surgeon during heart surgery have been repeated in the West. However it became clear that sedatives are often needed too, and that acupuncture can completely deaden the pain in some people only. Besides, there are not enough well-trained experienced acupuncturists to go around. For these reasons, as well as natural caution, it is not much used in the West except in dentistry and obstetrics. In both cases it has been shown to work with remarkable consistency.

We also know quite a lot about how acupuncture can deaden pain, as a result of recent research. There are natural painkillers, called endorphins, in our brain. They are there to reduce our pain feelings at critical times, for example in childbirth or in the thick of a fight. Acupuncture stimulates these brain endorphins, getting them to shut down pain over a much longer period than the usual four-hour morphine dose. Acupuncture works with the body's pain relief system; narcotics replace it. This is why the more you take of them the more you need them.

Acupuncture anaesthesia avoids the uncomfortable side effects and potential dangers of anaesthetics, it reduces pain after the operation, there is known to be less infection and tissue damage, much less shock to the system and the patient recovers more quickly. In fact acupuncture anaesthesia may be the only kind of anaesthesia possible in some patients who are suffering from shock, or are very weak, and cannot be given an operation using anaesthetic.

It is possible to substitute acupuncture for conventional drug anaesthesia in biopsies, minor surgery such as tonsillectomy, dentistry and obstetrics.

Under certain conditions replacing anaesthetics by acupuncture could be very important:

- If you are very weak or very ill
- If you have just had a heart attack
- If you have a weak liver
- If you have multiple allergies
- If you feel that the outcome of the operation will be poor

Do not worry about pain returning during the operation. The acupuncturist will constantly top up the anaesthesia by twirling the needles, and the anaesthetist will anyway be standing by.

Your acupuncturist will test you to check if you are anaesthetisable with acupuncture. If you are not, several acupuncture treatments before the operation can make you anaesthetisable with acupuncture. It will have the added bonus of improving your health and resistance to surgery.

It would be best to locate an anaesthetist who will be able to give you acupuncture anaesthesia at your request. However as they are thin on the ground you may need to shop around among your local acupuncturists for one who is able to induce anaesthesia. This should be done well before the date of the operation.

Acupuncture and postoperative healing: the problem of scarring

Scarring can be a disabling side effect of surgery, causing deep or superficial postoperative pain which can last for years. The pain clinics are full of such cases which are usually unrelieved by pain killers and require further operations and the cutting of nerves. The scar is like a geological fault. It consists of tough fibrous tissue which heals over the surgical disconnection between body parts. It can build up painful tensions, strains and blockages. It is likely that the majority of patients with persistent pain, tension, insomnia and stiffness after operations could be helped by acupuncture, which treats both the visible and the deep scars. The treatment often leads to a cathartic release of tension and emotion – the earthquake that releases the strain.

For example a 47-year-old housewife came to an acupuncturist reporting severe pain in the kidney area for twelve months, along with fatigue, weakness, and loss of hearing. The woman had a history of urogenital disorders. Her last two children were delivered by Caesarean. She had had a bladder repair operation and recently a hysterectomy. Her physician, an urologist and a gynecologist had all told her that there was nothing wrong with her and she should seek psychiatric help. So she went to an acupuncturist who pointed out the problem of scarring. When she was treated with acupuncture, the pattern of her pulses changed dramatically. After four scar treatments the patient described herself as feeling 30 years younger, full of energy, and resumed playing tennis.

Acupuncture can also stimulate healing and repair in the postoperative period. For example it has been discovered that if a leg is in a cast and wasting, acupuncture treatment on the *opposite* leg can reduce the wasting by 15 to 50 per cent. It works by redistributing energy. A similar effect to acupuncture can sometimes be obtained by therapeutic instruments which deliver pulses of electromagnetic energy. One type, called a 'TENS', has been found to heal deep tissue inflammation persisting after operations.

Shiatsu is acupuncture with the fingers, an Oriental massage therapy working with pressure on the acupuncture points. It is particularly suitable for postoperative patients with weak constitutions and, like massage, can be practiced in situations where an acupuncturist might not be welcomed. In this respect it is similar to reflexology (see below) with which it shares the ability to treat specific symptoms by pressure on defined points on the body. Shiatsu is particularly helpful after abdominal surgery which can upset the balance of the entire body. By working on points in the legs and arms, it can stimulate intestinal movement and normal organ function which is sluggish after surgery. You have to know the points so it is not suitable for self-care unless you learn it first.

Massage and reflexology after surgery

Massage is not just a pleasant way of spending an afternoon down by the pool. It is also serious therapeutic work. An experienced therapeutic massage will relax, realign, mobilize and revitalize tissues and organs. In a gentle but persistent manner the hands can be used to help healing, repair damage and improve the flow of energy and fluids. It is so obvious to use it after surgery that quite a few physiotherapists have added it to their repertoire. In hospitals in Russia and other CIS states, physiotherapists give each patient a good relaxing massage both before and after surgery.

Massage might also be of real value with critically ill patients in the Intensive Care Unit. For here the depersonalization, and deprivation are major problems and can inhibit health and recovery. On the other hand in the ICU massage should only be carried out by nurses or other medical staff, and care must be taken not to put the patient at risk, for example by disturbing blood clots. Recent British research examined 122 patients who had massage and aromatherapy while in Intensive Care. It concluded that massage was harmless and made the patients feel less anxious and more positive about their chances. At the Middlesex Hospital, one of the UK's leading medical centres, a clinical study was carried out with 100 cardiac patients on the day after surgery, while they were in the Intensive Care Unit, to test the effect of foot massage together with essential oils. The researchers found that during the 20 minutes massage, the patients felt soothed and relaxed, and their breathing slowed. For the next few days, the patients felt less anxiety, more calm, relaxed, and rested.

However issues of privacy and consent, and access through all the tubes and equipment can make it a little complex for nurses who can give massage in the ICU. Therefore if there is a nurse willing to do massage in the ICU, you should request it before the operation.

A massage can sometimes achieve things that you never imagined. For example, Avi Greenberg, an experienced therapeutic masseur, explains:

'After major surgery the blood is in the trunk. I move it to the periphery by massage and reflexology. I get the energy circulating around the body again. I bring warmth to the limbs, I push the lymph channels to get them to remove the waste, to bring the blood to the area of the surgery and clean it out, to start the process of healing and prevent infections. I use ambergris and rosemary oils to warm up the muscles and improve the circulation.'

Sometimes, after surgery, massage would be painful, or parts of the body should not be touched or are covered. Reflexology is a form of massage which works only on reflex points in the hands and feet, and it is obviously suitable in such cases. Through pressure on specific areas, the functioning of organs and repair of tissues can be encouraged. As Avi continues:

'I feel the surgical damage in the pressure points of the feet. But I do not work on the point related to the injured organ, such as the heart point after heart surgery. I work around the point, stimulating repair processes and circulation.'

Reflexology is gaining acceptability. It is used at the National Hospital for Nervous Diseases in London, especially with multiple sclerosis patients, and at the National Hospital for Sick Children, and at other hospitals in the UK and the US. However where it is not available or encouraged, it can be carried out by a reflexologist unobtrusively without requiring special permission from the staff.

Most surgical patients will be visited after surgery by a physiotherapist whose job it is to get your body moving again. She or he will try to reduce adhesions and stiffness, and exercise your body in order to restart doped organs. Physiotherapists used to be viewed as dragons that bore down on you before you were ready and forced you to move the painful parts. Today you may actually get a physiotherapist who will give you self-care exercises to do in bed, will help you with breathing; she may be able to give therapeutic massage. The physiotherapist is undoubtedly an ally in your path to recovery. However you may have to bring in some-one with professional skill in massage or reflexology in addition.

Homoeopathy and surgery

Little attention is usually paid by surgeons to reducing the shock of surgery and anaesthetics on the vital organs, and maintaining them in their best possible state. Homoeopaths feel that they have a special contribution to make in protecting the whole person during surgery, by using homoeopathic remedies. Homoeopathic remedies are minute, or invisible doses of natural materials which create healing reactions. The highly diluted or 'potentised' doses must be selected only by trained homoeopaths in response to your individual constitution and symptom picture.

At the Royal London Homoeopathic Hospital, homoeopathic remedies always accompany surgery. Frequently used remedies include:

- Aconite to protect against drug effects and shock.
- Phosphorus to stop bleeding.
- Bach Flower Remedies to reduce anxiety and stress.
- Arnica for shock and tissue damage.

Homoeopathy can also be used after surgery to deal with specific symptoms that may crop up. Dr E Roth, a well known medical homoeopath, described to me some examples: 'I have treated patients who have had surgery and come out of the anaesthesia with severe vomiting. This is treatable more easily homoeopathically than with conventional drugs. Healing after surgery is promoted with arnica or bellis perennis. The surgeon will usually say that he has never seen a patient recover so quickly.'

The kinds of symptoms treatable by homoeopathic remedies are unlike those usually treated by modern medicine. For example Professor Barriga, a well known surgeon-homoeopath at the Higino Perez Hospital in Mexico, would help the body adjust to fluid drips and transfusions, and control clotting and bleeding, by the use of arsenicum, pulsatilla or millefolium. To lift confusion and depression he might use gelsemium, hyoscyamus niger or coffea. He finds recovery is hastened by syphilinum, psorinum or aluminia and there are others to strengthen heart function, to sedate and calm, to reduce nausea, pain, infections, complications and so on.

As homoeopathic preparations are designed specifically for a set of symptoms expressed by a particular individual, you cannot normally just buy them off the shelf. You can however see a homoeopath beforehand for preparation for surgery, and then soon afterwards. Arnica and Bach Flower Remedies are exceptions in that they can be purchased for self-treatment of shock and distress. You can find these remedies in a homoeopathic first aid kit.

Herbs and essential oils in your surgical survival kit

A variety of problems can arise during or after surgery, from the serious (internal bleeding, toxemia, poor recovery, infected wounds) to the annoying but not dangerous (gastric problems, bruising, headaches, debility, insomnia). Herbs provide a wide range of therapeutic possibilities outside those of conventional medicine. If your ward doctor fails to deal with a particular problem that arises after surgery because he can't find the cause or the cure, or if the cure exists but the side effects of the drug concerned are too severe to tolerate, or if the problem is minor and you do not want to take more medical drugs for it, consider the option of herbs. However you should remember that it is the responsibility of the doctor to get you well. So normally you will add herbs to the treatment you are getting. You shouldn't substitute your own medicine for his without discussing it with him.

Herbs are taken as teas, tinctures, tablets, capsules or essential oils. It is always preferable in hospital to take them as teas or oils so as not to worry the medical staff with unusual tablets that they feel might interfere with their treatment. A herb tea can beneficially replace your usual hospital cuppa.

In suggesting herbs, we run in to the old problem that specific herbs, like other alternative remedies, should be prescribed specifically for each person. For example slow recovery might be due to poor absorption of nutrients (so take ginger, slippery elm), or poor digestion and metabolism (take gentian, dandelion root, chicory, fenugreek), or poor circulation in the relevant organs (rosemary, savory) or perhaps poor energy (take ginseng, damiana).

For this reason we can only give a general list of possibilities (as do most herb books) from which the right herbs should be selected on the basis of advice from a herbalist, knowledgeable friend or naturopath. Having said that if no other help is at hand, just try one or other of them as herb teas. (See also page 85 for general comments about using herbs in hospital, and page 94 for herbs to counter infections.)

Some preliminary investigations of the use of herbs along with surgery has taken place. In particular, a recent clinical study at St Bartholomews Hospital examined the ability of ginger powder to reduce post-operative nausea and vomiting. The chief anaesthesiologist there, Dr Bone, and his colleagues, reported that ginger was as good as conventional drugs against nausea. However the conventional tranquilizers that are used have noticeable side effects while ginger is harmless. In India a ginger-containing postoperative medicine called Gasex is used especially after stomach surgery. It reminds us of the great potential aromatic spices such as ginger, cinnamon and cloves have to stimulate the movement of the intestines, warm the body, and improve circulation and the absorption of food.

Panax notoginseng (Tienchi ginseng), a close relative of ginseng, is used in China to prevent blood clots, haemorrhage and bruising during surgery. In the traditional medical hospitals in China, many herbs are used to aid recovery and strength after surgery, and these still have not been studied in the West.

Essential oils of some of the plants described here can be used with great effect as part of post-operative massage by yourself or a masseur. Rosemary oil will aid circulation and relax tense muscles, and wheat germ oil will reduce inflammation. Comfrey oil or wheatgerm oil with extra vitamin E prevent scarring and can be massaged over operation scars once initial healing has taken place. Massage with oils of aromatic spices, basil, sage, or hyssop on the chest and torso to help overcome the effects of the anaesthetic. Neroli oil, the oil used in the study at the Middlesex

Hospital mentioned above, is soothing, and used for relaxation and the reduction of stress and anxiety.

Herbs for post-surgical symptoms

Symptoms	Herbs
Albuminurea	Goldenrod, juniper, broom, uva ursi.
Allergies	Liquorice, nettle, mullein, ephedra.
Anaemia after blood loss	Alfalfa, artichoke, chicory, dandelion, nettle, wheatgrass, kelp, lemon.
Anxiety/panic	Passionflower, valerian, skullcap.
Poor appetite	Gentian, sweet flag, angelica root, blessed thistle, centaury.
Bedwetting/poor urinary function	Uva ursi, heartsease, St John's wort, pumpkin seeds and seed oil, couch grass.
Poor circulation	Gingko biloba, cayenne, myrrh, rosemary.
Constipation	Aloe, rhubarb, senna, tamarin, linseed.
Bruising	Arnica, cajeput, hyssop, tea tree, St John's wort.
Slow recovery	American ginseng, chicory, damiana, fenugreek, rosemary, sage, savory.
Debility	Angelica, ginseng, damiana, liquorice, lobelia, oats, rosemary.
Slow healing of fractures	Comfrey, horsetail, nettle, parsley root.
Headache	Camomile, peppermint, rosemary, St John's wort, valerian, skullcap, willow bark.
Indigestion	Angelica, aniseed, caraway, ginger, peppermint, papaya.
Insomnia	Camomile, oats, melissa, skullcap, valerian.
Haemorrhage	Bayberry, golden seal, knotgrass, shepherd's purse, cramp bark, witch hazel.
Liver congestion and malfunction	Artichoke, milk thistle, boldo, chicory, dandelion, wormwood, tumeric, radish juice.
Nervous depression	Ginseng, basil, hyssop, jasmine, oats, sandalwood, St John's wort, valerian.
Shock	Arnica, basil, camphor, cayenne, ginseng, myrrh.

Symptoms	Herbs
Spasms and cramps	Catnip, cramp bark, hops, linden flowers, melissa, pennyroyal, sundew, skullcap.
Toxin accumulation	Alfalfa, asparagus, broom, dandelion, elder, garlic, parsley seed and root, yellow dock.
Vomiting and nausea	Aniseed, fennel seed, ginger, icelandic moss, ipecac, peppermint.
Slow wound healing	(internally) Astragalus, echinacea, tienchi ginseng, hyssop, snakeroot, sundew, red clover. (externally) Witch hazel, oak bark, comfrey, self-heal, aloe, cypress.

Which supplements should you add to your surgical survival kit?

After surgery you should get plenty of high-quality protein. Dietitians know this and will usually advise small tasty meals with concentrated protein foods. However there are also other special requirements for which supplementation may be needed: hospital institutional cooking is notorious for preserved and processed foods, and there is little attempt, even today, to provide a diet that contains enough vitamins, minerals, trace elements and essential fats for maximum health and recovery. This is discussed more fully in Chapter 3. Here we will remind you of the food factors that are needed to aid your post-operative recovery. Some of them, as advised previously, should begin to be taken some time before the operation.

If you are receiving sugar-saline drips, check that they are vita-minized, and if not, ask why. If you are not allowed to eat, the vitamins in the drip are especially important. In addition vitamin E capsules should be rubbed on externally as they are absorbed through the skin.

Vitamin C and bioflavonoids

Vitamin C is acknowledged to help in the healing of wounds, partly because it encourages the body to make collagen, the framework on which the tissues are built.

Surgery uses up vitamin C at a great rate and much more is needed by the white blood cells which clean up the mess and protect the body from infections. Over ten years ago the *British Medical Journal* stated that vitamin C should be given before surgery and on recovery, especially to the elderly. Your hospital should give it to you. If not, request it or bring it yourself.

What the hospital will not give to you is the partner to vitamin C which helps it work, the bioflavonoids. They are citrus peel extracts which minimize the oozing of capillaries and lessen the need for transfusion during surgery. The bioflavonoids also help vitamin C in collagen-building and tissue repair, so make sure you get it with your vitamin C (vitamin C + bioflavonoids are commonly available in one tablet). The dose is at least two grams per day.

Zinc

Zinc is one of the minerals which you should get in your diet but often don't. Even at the best of hospitals the food has been shown to provide less than the minimum daily requirement (MDR) of 15 mg of zinc for a healthy person. As a sick person, especially after surgery, you need much more, for zinc contributes to rapid wound repair and also supports the immune system. It is found in mineral-rich foods such as kelp, liver and yeast or can be bought as a food supplement.

B vitamins

The use of B vitamins is recommended for all hospital patients, mostly because of stress. Surgery exhausts the adrenal and other glands and can lead to salt imbalance, poor general functioning, exhaustion, infections and complications. Supplementation of B vitamins adds greatly to patient comfort after surgery. Nausea and vomiting after surgery, for example, can be prevented with vitamin B6. The dosage is given on page 82.

Vitamin E and scar prevention

Scar tissue is formed from inflammation and reduced blood supply when local blood vessels are damaged. Vitamin E increases the development of new vessels, prevents local inflammation and at the same time protects the glands and secretions necessary for recovery and repair. It has been used with great success in skin grafts and there is now good evidence that it prevents scars after surgery, including keloids (growth on scars) that form especially on dark skin. Scars have sometimes disappeared some time after surgery through consistently taking vitamin E. The scars are helped whether they are internal or external. For example scarring after bladder surgery can cause the bladder to contract so that it can't hold very much and urination is painful. The well-known nutritionist Adele Davis stated clearly that, 'In my 37 years of working in nutrition, I have seen nothing more spectacular than the role vitamin E plays in preventing ugly scars.' The dose is 500 IU before and after surgery. Those suffering from high blood pressure should start with 100 IU and move up over a week to the chosen dose. Vitamin E in wheat germ oil should be rubbed externally on scars.

Chapter Five

CANCER TREATMENTS: CHEMOTHERAPY AND RADIOTHERAPY

Sacred cows

Cancers are normal cells (the smallest units of living tissues) which have gone on a rampage. Drugs against cancer don't distinguish very well between 'wild' cancer cells and busy normal ones. Thus while attacking the cancer they also damage the lining of the stomach, the blood forming system and the immune system, leading to nausea, vomiting and loss of appetite and damage to the immunity.

The side effects of nausea and vomiting affect most people taking chemotherapeutic drugs, and one third of patients find them so unbearable that they have to stop treatment or lower the dosage. There are drugs against these side effects (for instance, nabilone) but they don't work very well and have their own side effects such as drowsiness and vertigo.

Chemotherapy also causes depression, tiredness and debility, hair falling out in about half of all cases (it regrows), and occasionally ulcers and nervous system problems. The side effects depend on the type of drug and the intensity of the treatment.

Radiation treatment kills cancer cells but, like the anticancer drugs, it also affects other normal cells. The side effects of radiotherapy are very similar to those of chemotherapy, with the added problem of local burns that can occur at the point of radiotherapy. However when radiotherapy is highly focused on the particular body region involved, there could be less general sickness and loss of immunity.

It is one of the tragic ironies of modern cancer treatment, therefore, that while attacking the cancer the treatments usually attack the body's own immune defences. Malignant tumors are continually changing and throw off seeds (metastases) which are difficult to detect and harder to treat. The patient needs every ounce of immunity during treatment, to mop up these seeds and to act against leftovers of the original tumor. Therefore by damaging immunity, chemotherapy and radiotherapy actually promote the spread of the cancer. In addition radiation and chemotherapy drugs are often themselves cancer-causing chemicals.

The end result of working against the patient's own resistance rather than with it is that battles are won but the war is lost. Sixty to eighty-five per cent of breast cancer patients will survive five years (depending on who's keeping the books) but only ten per cent will escape their cancer altogether. This is probably no more than the real cure rate of 100 years ago. For example, much trumpeted successes with drugs to add to surgery for breast cancer fizzled out when the figures were looked at more carefully. Short-term remissions were obtained, but at a heavy cost in side effects. Long term survival was not increased.

This means that the suffering from treatment side effects is often futile with 'many, many patients being given cytotoxics that cannot possibly help them', as Professor Timothy McElwain of the WHO advisory committee on Cancer Chemotherapy said at a meeting of the Society for Drug Research. Slowly, cancer experts are becoming less willing to give highly toxic anticancer drugs unless there is a reasonable chance of living rather longer because of them. This chance can be assessed by experience and by certain tests to measure how active the cancer is.

There is a whole herd of sacred cows involved with cancer treatment. For example, that it is urgent, that radiation and chemotherapy are always worth doing, that patients shouldn't be told about their disease, that diet has nothing to do with cancer treatment, that the patient's psychological condition is not relevant to the success of the treatment and that the side effects are a necessary evil and an unfortunate part of a life-saving effort. One by one these dogmas are being disproved. In this chapter we will consider mostly the last dogma. We will suggest some ways of deciding whether to accept such drastic treatments, we will look at some alternatives, and, above all, introduce some holistic ways of reducing the damage.

Cancer treatment choices

As conventional cancer treatment is usually drastic, and the disease is so serious, making decisions is difficult and taxing. Where cancer is concerned, the risk versus benefit of any particular treatment option can be rephrased: how much will it reduce the quality of my life and how much will it increase the length of my life. You should ask the oncologist (cancer specialist) to give you his assessment of quality versus quantity. If there is no clear answer, it may be better not to have the treatment. No medical treatment is *not* the same as doing nothing. Don't forget that there are alternatives to conventional medical treatment for cancer, the so-called 'gentle' approach, which is briefly described below.

The need for full and balanced information is obviously even more important and helpful in the case of cancer than where less serious decisions have to be made. It is unfortunate, therefore, that doctors are particularly likely to pull the wool over your eyes in relation to cancer. This is partly because they themselves find it difficult to cope with the emotional intensity of clear statements. It is partly because they need to believe in unrealistic expectations in order to keep the entire cancer-treatment machine rumbling along. Sometimes they simply don't know or they may feel that the patient doesn't want to know. Therefore they will typically downplay the disease, or lie about it to both patients and family, or worse, to the patient only while telling the truth to everyone else. According to a recent poll in New York, if you were dying only one in four doctors would tell you. Be aware of the temptation everyone feels to avoid the truth. Even in the very worst case, where the doctors would give a patient only a short time to live, knowing the truth allows the patient to question toxic, hopeless treatments and explore gentler ways to treat himself.

In the case of cancer it is necessary to know your chances, that is, the statistics. Before accepting a treatment strategy check on the five-year survival figures for the relevant cancer, check if they have changed in the last ten years. This will give you an independent view of how successful conventional medicine is likely to be in your case and help you to judge whether it is worth it. Check the statistics, if you can, of the department where you will be treated and compare them with the national statistics.

Oncologists are always in dispute about treatments among themselves, and always trying out new treatment combinations which have not necessarily been fully evaluated. Some believe in the psychological aspect and will work with counsellors and psychologists. Others think that cancer is entirely due to random factors and patient weaknesses are humbug. Some oncologists will be prepared automatically to give highly toxic drugs believing that the ends always justify the means. Others will not do so. For example removal of the entire breast of women with diagnosed breast cancer used to be the norm until it was discovered that removal of the lump only ('lumpectomy') gave the same five-year survival figure.

For these reasons it is very important that you choose a specialist who has a long experience of the disease. Treatment by doctors who are less experienced is more likely to be by the 'current formula' leading to more side effects for less benefit. Specialist doctors should be able to assess your progress more sensitively and on that basis decide on the most worthwhile treatments. Second opinions are essential. If this results in a conflict between two equally authoritative views, it is usually better to choose the opinion that advises the less drastic treatment, given the current confusions.

The top cancer specialists may wish to try out new treatments. If these are better methods of targeting drugs, or new safer drug combinations, or immunological and unconventional methods such as hyperthermia (high temperature) treatment, they may be very helpful. But be wary of accepting treatments in which side effects are not established or those in which the benefits are questionable but irreversible damage is done to organs or immunity.

It has been clearly demonstrated that those people who have a fighting, positive, active attitude to their disease are more likely to survive it whereas those who give up hope do not survive as long. 'Those who survived the longest were real troublemakers,' said Dr Bernard Fox, Professor of Psychiatry at Boston University Medical School. 'They fought with their doctors, sought alternative opinions and methods of treatment. They refused to relinquish hope and struggled to survive.' It is now beginning to be accepted that there is no such thing as 'spontaneous regression' which is a medical admission of ignorance about cancers which disappear by themselves. The cancers tend to disappear in people who have faith, independence, emotionally transforming experiences and active involvement in their disease. In a word, people who are really determined to live have a fighting chance to get over the disease.

Alternative cancer treatments

Like all natural medicine, alternative cancer therapies are based on self-healing and purification or detoxification. They are developments of the naturopathic view that cancers arise through dietary impurities, weak immunity, and psychological stress. The cures work by encouraging the self-healing ability of the body to remove the cancer naturally. They use multivitamin supplements, strict dietary control, counselling, mental imagery or self-hypnosis, art therapy, spiritual healing, immunological support (through herbal and organ extracts or the induction of fevers), herbs and so on. The methods are described in books such as *A Time To Heal, A Cancer Therapy – Results of 50 Cases, Cancer: Your Life, Your Choice,* and *Loving Medicine* (see Appendix 1).

Most patients arrive at alternative treatment centres after failed or unbearable medical treatment. Alternative practitioners claim that all these patients will have a better life and better death, and that some will live longer than expected, and this seems a reasonable claim. However it would be wrong to raise false expectations. Alternative methods are not a panacea. Thus to go to a counselling group, or become a vegetarian should not be seen as a substitute for deep, serious and committed treatment whether conventional or alternative. The diet is seen as assisting, not re-placing, treatment.

Although doctors won't accept that methods such as imagery can treat the disease, they are interested in these same methods when used to make patients feel more comfortable and reduce side effects of treatment. There are laws in several countries, including the UK, against alternative practitioners claiming they can treat cancer. The famous Bristol Cancer Centre had to change its name to Bristol Cancer Help Centre and when Prince Charles visited there was a storm of protest from the conventional doctors and their representatives. Yet you will be able to find doctors who are willing to try parts of 'unorthodox' therapies, such as hypnosis, if it can reduce pain or help patients to accept the orthodox treatment.

It is worth remembering that even if you choose to look into the 'gentle' approach, you do not need to abandon conventional medicine. A recent survey of 356 patients using alternative cancer treatments found that only 15 per cent completely rejected the conventional methods and 60 per cent used both at the same time. Researchers have concluded that 'Many intelligent and resourceful patients are integrating established and alternative therapies in their personal search for a treatment "programme" that makes sense to them and fits their needs...'

The methods can be quite demanding, needing persistence and will. There is work to be done – preparing juices and special foods, taking nutritional supplements, going through counselling. It can also be a very rewarding and fulfilling experience. Some patients are absolutely ready for this. They are determined to live and cure themselves, and are frustrated at the passivity demanded by con-ventional treatment. Others would rather leave it to the doctor, as they don't feel up to it. It is a personal choice. However the gentle approach can give you the encouragement to go further. One woman wanted to treat herself using natural therapies, but didn't have the strength. She went on a supervised grape juice fast for a while simply in order to develop the energy and determination to fight her cancer, which she managed to do very successfully.

Hypnosis, imagery and other methods of controlling side effects and empowering treatment

'I was having a long course of chemotherapy for leukemia and the nausea and vomiting got worse and worse. I couldn't eat or keep a meal down when in hospital and I was sick as soon as I saw the nurse who was to give me treatments. Drugs didn't work so I called in a hypnotist. He relaxed me but I 'saw through' the procedure and it didn't help. A psychotherapist was invited by my doctor, and I told him that I was sceptical but was happy for him to try.

He immediately asked me to focus on my sensations of breathing, and I let his voice come over me. He asked me to feel comfortable and relaxed and to let him know by signs how deeply relaxed I felt. I was encouraged to enjoy and revel in the feelings. Then he gently woke me out of them. I don't remember very clearly what happened in my next session but I was told that after reaching a deep level of relaxation the various parts of chemotherapy treatment – travelling to hospital, meeting the nurse, receiving the injection – were described by the hypnotist with the same suggestion of comfort. I was asked to let him know by raising a finger if any of these events disturbed my comfort, and, amazingly, none of them did.

After the second session of hypnosis I didn't vomit any more and by the end of the week I was eating a full meal. The vomiting and nausea never came back.'

This is a rather typical case, reported by Dr M Hoffman in the *American Journal of Clinical Hypnosis*. For the use of hypnotherapy to control the side effects of cancer treatment is a great success story. In the late 1960s and early 1970s cancer treatment centres were exploring the use of hypnosis to control pain, and researchers noticed that it also reduced or prevented certain side effects of chemotherapy and radiotherapy. When they tried it with patients for whom the antivomiting drugs didn't work they usually lost their nausea and vomiting, as well as a good deal of anxiety. Moreover patients returned to themselves, gaining confidence so that healing could begin. Clinical studies that have been published in the last few years have made it clear that progressive relaxation itself, as we described in the last chapter, is able to reduce the symptoms of nausea and vomiting. However hypnosis and the use of imagery go one step further and achieve correspondingly better results.

Dr Newton, summarizing his eight-year experience using hypnosis with 283 cancer patients noted: *The absolutely indispensable part of our work is the patients' experiencing the most profound quiet on a regular daily basis.* Virtually all of his patients had experienced a great increase in the quality of life. The survival times of those patients who already had spreading cancer (advanced metastases) of breast, bowel and lung were about three times longer than national statistics.

Hypnosis cannot cure cancer. Yet there is little doubt that climbing from a depressed well of despair to an independent, positive, living determination can result in remission. Psychological strength of this kind helps the immune system attack the cancer. A study at the University of Pittsburgh, to cite one example of the evidence, found that cancer patients who were compliant, listless, without energy and vigor and were resigned to their disease had much lower levels of cancer-attacking white cells ('natural killer' cells) than those with a more positive attitude. In other words, hypnosis and relaxation techniques clearly reduce the side effects of treatment and may also so change the patient's state of mind that the body's ability to fight the cancer itself is strengthened.

Here is a case which illustrates this effect, reported by Dr Dempster and colleagues in the *International Journal of Clinical and Experimental Hypnosis*:

'A young woman with Hodgkins Disease was receiving nitrogen mustard and her side effects were so severe that the specialists were just about to stop chemotherapy altogether. The hypnotist induced a light trance and asked her to pick a colour and then to imagine flames dancing in a fireplace. The flames were all kinds of colours which eventually coalesced into the colour she chose. She was taught to imagine sinking into this colour whenever she wanted to carry out self-hypnosis. She was given suggestions that the pain and inflammation, the nausea and the other symptoms would go, and they did. And as hypnosis continued she found that she could take part in life again. She travelled, completed her college degree, started some voluntary work, and could live fully during the time she had, which was longer than predicted.'

Children often enter altered states of consciousness naturally, and hypnosis is much easier than with adults. Yet children can suffer terribly from the fear, pain and discomfort of cancer treatments. It is thus essential that hypnosis or imagery is used with children receiving toxic cancer treatments. It is usually successful. For example, all children receiving cancer treatments at the Minneapolis Children's Health Centre who have unpleasant medical side effects are referred for hypnosis and imagery. The techniques used are very flexible to allow the children to suggest and develop their own themes. In one case (reported in the *American Journal of Pediatric Hematology/Oncology*) an eight-year-old girl was under treatment for acute lymphoblastic leukemia. She had to have painful bone marrow examinations, and was taught pain control by using 'switches' to switch off the pain at places in her body. Before the next bone marrow examination the therapist induced a light trance and suggested that she turn off her pain switches over the bone. The oncologist came. 'Hand-in-hand, she and the oncologist walked to the treatment room. She had no pre-medication. She climbed on to the table and the examination was completed in two minutes with no anaesthesia...she walked out with her doctor, returned to her room and, within a few minutes seemed happily engrossed in games and colouring.'

A study reported in the *British Journal of Clinical and Experimental Hypnosis* used 'nausea management training' to help patients. This is a technique of reexperiencing the nausea while relaxed and under hypnosis, and then receiving suggestions and triggers to reduce it. The technique worked well, so much so that Dr Ashley Conway, reviewing this study, could not help stating: 'What is remarkable, and appalling, is that this kind of support is not widely available to patients in this country.' Clearly patients will have to demand it.

Healing is another option. A boost of healing energy during treatment can protect the immunity and normal body processes. It can also help to eliminate lingering after-effects of the treatment. It is especially effective at removing the weary tension that may follow radiotherapy or chemotherapy. Healers have reported success with patients who suffer from partial paralysis due to the irradiation of a nerve during cancer treatment. The healer will focus on the nerve and help it to work again, in combination with both imagined and actual physiotherapy.

However healing itself has short term effects. To build on this you should work with the healer on self-healing techniques and developing a positive healthy attitude. Three quarters of the people who come to see Matthew Manning, possibly Britain's best-known healer, have cancer, and most request help with treatment effects. He stresses that if you believe that the treatment is helpful it will be. Healing should become part of a process, so that the energy, vitality and relief given by the healer is transformed into the inner drive to be well. Healers often teach self-hypnosis to patients and encourage them to look at why they became ill. This works better if the healer and client are 'resonating' on the same wavelength, that is, they communicate well and feel good with each other. Bear this in mind when selecting a healer as with any therapist.

Acupuncture and acupressure can help to control treatment symptoms. This has been known for some time in the west because of the watchful eye on China, in which acupuncture has been routine as a procedure to help reduce pain, nausea and other adverse effects of medical procedures. Now there is a track record in Western countries too. Every acupuncturist I spoke to had some experience with patients that came to them for supportive help during a course of chemotherapy or radiotherapy or similarly drastic procedures. There is good reason too. For acupuncture rebalances and restores the balance of function in the organs, which has been thrown off by the treatment. Acupuncture is also known to act on brain hormones called enkephalins, which are known to be the substances which can control both pain and vomiting. The late Professor John Dundee, of the University Hospital at Leeds, UK, has carried out many full-scale clinical studies of the use of acupuncture to control chemotherapy – induced nausea and vomiting. In one example, 130 patients received acupuncture at the P6 wrist point. 93 per cent reported complete absence or improvement of nausea and/or vomiting, with 63 per cent reporting no sickness at all for at least eight hours after the chemotherapy. Though the patients in this study were also taking conventional drugs against vomiting, the results were far better than were achieved by the conventional drugs alone. There is therefore good reason to include a skilled acupuncturist in the supporting team during cancer treatments.

Imagery and visualization

Images are very often used as part of hypnosis. They can also be an important self-help technique on their own, bringing specific beneficial effects to body, mind and spirit. Imagery is well illustrated by the oft-quoted case of a young haemophiliac who was bleeding profusely. While the doctor was preparing emergency aid the bleeding stopped. The astonished doctor asked the child 'What happened?' He said, 'Oh, I put some super-glue on it.'

The specific use of imagery to treat cancer has been pioneered by the Simontons in the US. Their method typically involves imagining, in a state of relaxation, the cancer being attacked and cleaned out by the body's defences. For example: 'Your white blood cells are fish swimming in and eating up the grayish cancer cells. Project this image as if it were on a screen that you're viewing in your mind's eye. When you have that image very clear then become one of the fish and lead the rest of the shoal into the attack. After this, feel yourself engaging in activities you would pursue if you were healthy. Picture yourself at the healthiest time in your life and create images of the present, feeling just that way.'

More to the point, images can be used to support medical treatment, making it more effective and less harmful. You can imagine chemotherapy as chemicals dismantling the tumor and leaving normal tissues unharmed, or the radiotherapy as a great white healing sun that cleanses and cures with its rays. This can empower treatment to do its job, and even the side effects are seen as the medicine working, and therefore an encouraging sign. 'The balder you get the better – for every hair that falls a cancer cell dies. It is just death followed by regeneration', is how one patient put it.

Such images, by giving power to the treatment to do its job, get you completely involved in the treatment. You 'own' your treatment. This positive, active attitude gives you faith that you will get better and helps to mop up side effects on the way. An artist Gillian told me how she would visualize the radiation as a big dragon's eye, powerful and inspiring. When she needed a mask to protect her pituitary glands from radiation damage she made one herself, decorating it beautifully and covering it with feathers. It helped her welcome the treatment. Her hospital, in Hackney, London, ran visualization classes which she joined. She feels not only that she has gained an extra 18 months, but that she has lived more in that 18 months than in her whole life before.

Roger Parsons, another ex-patient, told us how after he had been diagnosed as having cancer he went down to London, to the Royal Marsden Hospital, as he wanted to be treated by the top specialists. He started chemotherapy there and at the same time went to the Bristol Centre who gave him dietary advice which he was able to pursue while staying in hospital. He cut out all fats, sugar, salt, meat, preservatives, and caffeinated drinks. He ate raw foods, grains, seeds, nuts, fruit and goat's cheese. 'I started relaxation and visualization with tapes. A sister at the hospital used to go with me to the Day Room and play the tapes. I fell asleep and she did the exercises! Nevertheless I felt sure it helped me relax and gain confidence. In order to remove the fear of chemotherapy I sat up all night with another patient, talking him through his fears and losing my own in the process. I agreed to chemotherapy only when I felt sure it would work. When I received the drugs I watched them going into my body, and I loved them, knowing they were doing me good. I did have side effects, but they were minimal. I shaved my hair off to preempt it falling by itself. During the treatment I would visualize the cancer being excreted from my body every time I went to the toilet. I also spent long hours every day gazing off-centre at the sun, as I had heard somewhere that this was a support for the immune system. I took vitamins, especially vitamin C, and continued with my special diet. I was glad to stay in the hospital as it enabled me to focus exclusively on getting better.'

After some months metastases in his lungs disappeared, and doctors removed the original tumor – it was 'dead', encysted, and he is cured.

The way to use images specifically to reduce side effects is illustrated by the case of a young girl, Judy, who used a very interesting image during her radiotherapy. She imagined that her hair was like coconut matting and that each of her hairs was tied under the scalp with a little knot, so that it was impossible for them to fall out. She said that it worked.

Both hypnosis and imagery or visualization need to be strong and deep. They work by unlocking the energies deep inside you and the more you submerge yourself in the imagery or in hypnosis, the better the effect. This does not mean that the pictures have to be vivid, because it has been found that some people with less clear visualizations can be helped and others with very vivid visualizations are not. But it must involve all of you. If it is superficial it will simply act like relaxation – helpful to relieve anxiety but without the more specific effects we have described.

It is essential to obtain expert guidance in order to get deep enough in these techniques and to select those images which are meaningful and appropriate for your life and personality. For example the more aggressive attacks on cancer cells in the Simonton visualizations may have been suitable for some of their patients, but others found it too warlike. Erica, a 60-year-old woman who has herself become a healer, felt that her cancer needed love and attention.

'The cells grow and become too big because they are seeking attention. If I give it to them they don't eat so much. I feel compassion to both my good tissues and my cancer tissues. They are both me and mine. When I had radiotherapy, I imagined myself going through my body as a garden, giving water and good things to the good plants and taking care of the weeds too.'

A new study at St Mary's Hospital in London carried out by a team of researchers under Professor Priest showed that relaxation and imagery were effective in improving mood and reducing stress during radiotherapy for breast cancer. As we mentioned above, imagery with relaxation was found to be more effective than relaxation alone. 'Often the images made the patient smile, at a time when smiles were perhaps few and far between.' They also preferred a more peaceful pleasant scene of the patient's choice as a suitable image, since it is a resource already within each of us. The more aggressive visualizations of the cancer being attacked may also leave a discouraging sense of failure if it doesn't seem to be working.

Colette, an inspiring teacher of visualization, insists that her main role is to select an image that is deeply meaningful for each person: 'the image must be extremely startling to upset the patient's balance momentarily. It strikes. Then they do it intensely and briefly three or four times a day. The image actually comes from the patient, from their biography, I only induce it.' She told the story of an elderly woman with a brain tumor who couldn't move her arms. She shocked her by saying that at her age she wouldn't teach her gradually to regain movement. She would teach her flamenco! The imaginary flamenco and another visualization of cooking green peas and then eating them with a fork helped her regain a good deal of arm and wrist movement.

You should receive hypnosis, or training in imagery, several times to become familiar with the technique and build a rapport with the therapist. You will then normally be taught to do it yourself and be given a tape to help if conditions are disturbing. If you do your 'homework' regularly it will provide you with an instant inner sanctuary. During uncomfortable medical treatment you can take a few slow steady breaths and, with imagery, quickly slip into a quiet state of relaxation which will continue until you fall asleep or become disturbed. If you are disturbed a symptom such as vomiting can immediately return. However the homework will enable you to regain control, and reabsorb yourself in the images.

Diet during cancer treatments

If you ask a cancer specialist which diet would help his treatment, he would probably answer merely: 'a good one'. 'To be unable to give a satisfactory response to this question is not only embarrassing for the physician, but it is also dangerous for the patient', complained one cancer specialist.

Only in holistic medicine is diet used instead of, or together with, the drastic cancer treatments of chemotherapy, radiotherapy and surgery. The diets are intended to detoxify the body completely, restore the work of the organs and the immune system, and expose the tumor to attack by the body's white blood cells. The diets are best used as part of a complete natural system of cancer treatment involving also enemas, herbal medicines, fasts, exercise, psychotherapy and so on. This natural system works better when the body and immunity have not been damaged by chemotherapy and radiotherapy. However it is accepted that for many patients the best option is to choose both conventional and holistic treatments. In that case the diet is intended to add to the conventional treatment by improving the quality and length of life, and preventing the side effects of treatment. There are, in fact, a great many cases where diets have helped prevent the destructive effects of cancer treatments. A study with 56 patients found that nine out of ten of those given an enriched natural diet improved after radiotherapy, compared with five out of ten on a normal diet.

The most well known diet is *naturopathic*, pioneered by Dr Hans Moolenburgh and Max Gerson (see Appendix 1). Its main components are:

- No sugar, fats, alcohol, coffee, tea, tobacco, food preservatives or additives and almost no salt. This eliminates the stress of further contamination of the body.
- High-fibre vegetarian diet with added liver extract. The vegetables should be young, fresh and organically grown on good soil. About 20 per cent of the diet should be raw vegetables especially carrots, radish, sprouts, beets, greens, cucumber, parsley, onions and dandelion tops. Cooked

vegetables should be minimally cooked or steamed in stainless steel or enamel saucepans.
- Only cold-pressed oils, especially sesame or olive oil.
- Minimal starches, depending on the condition of the patient, derived from seeds, oatmeal or muesli and brown rice.
- Protein-rich seeds such as pulses, sesame, buckwheat, all nuts, pumpkin and sunflower seeds, mung beans, and apricot kernels (which are therapeutic).
- Spring or mineral water. No chlorinated, fluoridated or recycled water.
- Fruit. Dried or fresh.
- Vegetables and fruit should also be prepared in the form of total juices, at least 1 litre (2 pints) per day.
- Garlic. Kelp. Yeast.
- Raw milk products, particularly yoghurt and kefir, at certain stages of the treatment only.
- A number of organ extracts and nutritional supplements.

Not all of the above are permitted at the early stages of treatment which might involve exclusively juices and organ extracts. Preliminary reports show that provided patients receive counselling for emotional health in parallel with the diets for physical health, there are excellent chances of outliving all expectations.

Dr Peter Lechner at the largest hospital in Austria, the Landeskrankenhaus, studied patients with advanced cancer of the digestive system whom he treated with the Moolenburgh and Gerson diet. He reports that his diet patients were in excellent general condition even in very advanced cases, and were surviving longer than all predictions. He was mostly able to replace narcotics with aspirin-type painkillers. None of the patients needed tranquilizers, sedatives or similar drugs, and he reports that not one of the diet patients needed to have their chemo- and radiotherapy reduced because of side effects. These patients 'were protected against depressed blood counts, loss of hair, depressed liver function, and other well known negative side effects of chemotherapy'.

Another dietary system that has helped many cancer patients over their treatment is *macrobiotics*. It is a purifying dietary system based on Oriental concepts of harmony and balance. It involves balancing pure natural foods, particularly brown rice, fresh specially prepared vegetables, dried pulses and beans, seaweeds, buckwheat and Japanese soya products such as miso, according to the constitution and condition of each person. It holds to the prohibitions of sugar, alcohol, and so on described above, but does not add all the special food factors and supplements found in the Gerson diet. The diet must be continually altered depending on the patient's progress through the disease, and therefore needs to be supervised by an expert. Details of this diet are given in Michio Kushi's inspiring book on the anti-cancer diet (see Appendix 1).

We talked to Diana, a small, strong-willed 46-year-old woman who first noticed a lump on her breast in September 1981, which was not diagnosed as cancer until 1984, by which time it had ulcerated and spread. She underwent six weeks of intensive radiotherapy even though the radiotherapist felt it might be too late, and was given six months to live. She started a strict, guided macrobiotic diet at the same time. She didn't feel sick or tired throughout the treatment which she was told was exceptional. After radiotherapy the breast healed completely. The radiotherapist was very pleased and said that he 'had seen it happen once before'. She refused surgery and concentrated on her diet, with her sister cooking it and going on it herself to encourage her. Though she lost a lot of weight, which worried the doctors, she felt she was getting better and managed a second course of radiotherapy without any side effects other than superficial burns. She is not through the wood yet, but at present has no detectable metastases. She looks well, with bright eyes and an enthusiastic, lively presence.

Vitamins and dietary supplements

The way vitamins can protect you against diagnostic radiation has already been discussed in Chapter 2. Since radiotherapy may use doses 1000 times greater, the need for vitamins is even more obvious. Both radiotherapy and chemotherapy drastically deplete the body of vitamins which need to be made up. And vitamins not only protect against side effects, but may also help the struggle of the immunity against the cancer.

Vitamin C
In 1977 Professor Linus Pauling, Nobel Laureate and one of the greatest scientific figures of our time, shocked the medical world by announcing that vitamin C treatment can prolong the lifetime of cancer patients, alleviate their suffering and help in the side effects of treatments. He based this on Dr Ewan Cameron's research on 100 cancer patients given vitamin C at the Vale of Leven Hospital in Scotland, who appeared to survive four times longer than average. A furious scientific debate ensued, which still continues. The current view is that when vitamin C is given along with chemotherapy or radiotherapy it can make the treatment more effective and less toxic. For example, scientists at Wake Forest University in the US found that when the anticancer drugs vinblastine and vincristine are given along with vitamin C, weight and hair loss were avoided. The treatment did not lose any effectiveness. Other evidence shows that anticancer drugs such as 5-FU or methotrexate are rendered more effective by giving vitamin C during treatment.

Vitamin C is acting as an 'anti-oxidant' that is, it protects against the free radical damage caused by radiation, as discussed in Chapter 2. It also helps to neutralise toxins, protect and enhance the immunity, and support the adrenal glands in their fight against stress. The dose is large, five to ten grams per day, and should be taken on the advice of a nutritional expert.

Vitamin E and selenium
Both of these food factors act as antioxidants in the body's damage-control systems. Vitamin E, for example, has been shown to enhance the effect of anticancer drugs such as vincristine, and prevent damage to heart, skin and lungs that tends to occur when the drugs adriamycin and bleomycin are used. Selenium backs up vitamin E and has been successfully tried as part of cancer treatment. The dose of vitamin E is around 600 IU per day, and selenium 225 micrograms per day.

Vitamin A
The retinoids, a group of substances which includes vitamin A, are now known to be among the most effective cancer protective

substances in nature. They are also widely recognized to be helpful in supporting the immunity and exposing cancer cells to treatment. The dose is around 30,000 IU per day of vitamin A (beta carotene).

B vitamins
They work in the liver to remove the toxins created during treatment. Together with vitamins A and C, they also prevent damage to the immune system, helping to remove dead cells and prevent the cancer spreading. These vitamins can also prevent the tiredness and debility that result from cancer treatments.

A study some years ago at the Montefiore Hospital in New York compared patients who received intensive radiotherapy with and without yeast supplements. Those who took three tablespoons of yeast starting a week before treatment experienced far fewer side effects. The most important vitamin for protection against nausea and vomiting is B6, but pantothenic acid and folic acid are both useful in preventing toxicity. Take around 50 milligrams of each of the B vitamins, in the form of B complex.

A high-dose vitamin regimen should be commenced at least one week before the start of radiotherapy or chemotherapy. It is very hard to give an absolute dosage guide because it varies from person to person depending on the state of the liver, body weight, condition of the disease and so on. Therefore it is important to seek the advice of a holistically-minded doctor who will guide you. At the same time check with the doctor giving you chemotherapy if there are any special nutritional requirements associated with the particular chemotherapeutic drug he is giving you. For example cis-platin has been shown to deplete zinc and magnesium because of its effects on the kidneys, and methotrexate prevents calcium and magnesium from being absorbed from food.

Preventing and treating radiation burns and hair losses

Excellent results have been obtained with vitamin E to *prevent* radiation burns, a frequent and very unpleasant side effect of radiotherapy. The usual problem is that the burns are not given a chance to heal because of repeated radiation treatment. Vitamin E prevents the burning in the first place,and greatly diminishes the pain and subsequent scarring of the area. Vitamin E in wheat germ oil should be applied liberally to the area before and after every treatment and once or twice a day in the interval. If it is available only in capsules pierce them with a pin and apply the contents.

Aloe vera gel is probably the best material for the *cure* of radiation burns if they do occur. Japanese survivors of the atomic bombs who applied aloe vera gel to radiation burns healed more rapidly and with less scarring than those that did not. There is relief from pain and inflammation, and more rapid regrowth of tissues. Aloe can dry the skin so other skin care agents should be added. A 55-year-old woman from Oxford had a mastectomy followed by eight weeks of radiation treatment twice a week. She was in considerable pain from the burns which didn't heal. A friend of mine gave her little pots of aloe vera plants to have at home. Morning and evening she would break a leaf and apply the juice. From the very first day, she said, the pain was reduced, the skin looked better and she was able to give up painkillers.

The American International Hospital in Illinois has found that an 'ice bonnet' placed on the scalp 15 minutes before chemotherapy and radiotherapy and left on 30 minutes afterwards, will stop hair loss. Even if it does fall out during cancer treatment the hair grows back, sometimes quite luxuriantly.

Shingles and viral diseases

The inhibition of immunity caused by cancer treatments leaves the patient extremely vulnerable to infections during the period of treatment. Usually patients are given gamma-globulin injections to improve resistance, and any onset of an infection is quickly treated by antibiotics. But shingles and viral infections can occur at this time, and there is little that can be done apart from giving painkillers. If a viral infection does occur, take five grams per day of vitamin C. Vitamin E oil (see above) is quite effective when rubbed on shingles and it should also be taken internally. Herbs can also be very useful, but to get the best out of them, it would be advisable to consult a herbalist or naturopath. For nerve inflammations you can use aconite, rue, skullcap, St John's wort, and for viral infections you could use echinacea, St John's wort, burdock or golden seal.

Herbal and homoeopathic remedies against treatment symptoms

Where there is an existing herbal tradition it would be unthinkable to allow people to go through the devastating experience of cancer treatment without calling on the rich resources of plant medicines to help them. In Switzerland many family doctors will automatically send cancer patients for herbal treatment of chemotherapy symptoms such as poor appetite, tiredness, nausea, vomiting, skin irritations and liver upset. There is no single prescription for these side effects – different herbalists will prescribe different herbs depending on their experience and the particular symptoms involved. The symptomatic use of herbs is ancient, well tried, and often remarkably successful.

Aloe vera
This is an important part of natural cancer treatment, taken internally in prescribed amounts. It can protect the intestines and restore their function if they are affected by chemotherapy and radiotherapy. Like many bitter or aromatic herbs, it also stimulates the appetite and digestion. Aloe vera can be combined with classical bitter herbs such as angelica root or rhubarb and these 'bitters' are available from herbal suppliers. Alternatively you can take aloe vera by itself as a juice or in capsules.

Seaweed products, Irish/Icelandic moss, linseed (flaxseed), slippery elm bark
All these materials protect the digestive system by soothing it with a mucilaginous coating. Alginate, from seaweeds, is sometimes given to people who have been accidentally exposed to radiation. One research project investigated what happened when an extract of the seaweed *Digenia simplex* was given to 162 patients who

received radiation for bone cancer. It was found that it prevented nausea, loss of appetite, debility and some pain. Seaweeds such as kelp can also reduce swellings in the lymph glands. The dose is quite high – around ten to fifteen grams per day.

Spices
Spices are utilized in the Indian Ayurvedic tradition to clear toxins from the body and to restore normal function. The pungent spices, particularly ginger, are particularly effective at restoring proper blood supply and organ function, particularly of the digestive system. Ginger is able to both stimulate and soothe the digestive system, and help to prevent it reacting to the toxins of chemotherapy by nausea. Several clinical studies have shown that ginger is the best of anti-nausea herbs in a number of common situations such as motion sickness, morning sickness in pregnancy and postoperative nausea. Clinical studies with patients receiving chemotherapy are limited as yet. However one double blind clinical study at the University of Birmingham, Alabama, USA, demonstrated that ginger was effective at preventing chemotherapy induced nausea, but not vomiting.

Marijuana
Cannabis has been discovered to be effective at reducing nausea and vomiting during chemotherapy. In the last few years a half dozen synthetic drugs have been developed based on the cannabis components and one, nabilone, is in general use in the UK. It seems absurd that the herb cannabis, which is cheap, natural, safe and well tried, is illegal; not even doctors can prescribe it without permission whereas its main ingredient chemical, requiring millions of dollars to develop, and with known and unknown side effects, is described as a welcome discovery. In any event, cannabis itself can be eaten before chemotherapy, and besides anti-nausea effects, may help reduce pain. The dosage should be established by consultation.

Herb teas
Strong teas of peppermint or one teaspoonful of ginger (preferably fresh), combined with crushed seeds of aniseed and fennel, are effective at reducing nausea and vomiting.

Herbal cancer treatments

There are no sure cancer cures, whether conventional or alternative, and it is our purpose to discuss the side effects of treatment rather than the treatment itself. Nevertheless I should mention that there are herbs that can be used to help treat and expel tumors. They include violet, chapparal, pokeroot, Pau d'arco and red clover. Such herbs should only be used under professional advice.

Homoeopathic Remedies

These can be used to deal with specific symptoms as they occur. But they must be prescribed for *you* by a homoeopath after your individual homoeopathic diagnostic symptom picture has been established. Homoeopathic remedies against unwanted symptoms are based on the materials that create the same symptoms in the healthy. For this reason homoeopaths have used highly diluted preparations of radium bromide, uranium nitrate or cadmium sulphate against radiation sickness, and phosphorus or fluoric acid to help cure radiation burns. I received a letter from a woman in Wales who had had 25 radiation treatments. After the eighteenth the doctors had to halt treatment because her sensitive skin suffered from burns. A homoeopath gave her cantharis six times a day. A week later she went for the rest of her treatments which were so successful that the nurse remarked about her tough skin, and the radiotherapist said he had never known such healing.

Protecting your immunity during cancer treatments

The hidden side effects of radiotherapy and chemotherapy, which may be more serious than the obvious ones, are on the immune system. The immune system may suffer severe damage and need strong support. The best way to protect and encourage the immunity is to take Chinese herbs. It is ironic that Oriental medicine has developed a wide range of immune-supporting remedies, just as Western medicine has a wide range of immune-destroying remedies.

Three important immune-supporting Oriental herbal remedies are astragalus, ligusticum and codonopsis. Astragalus root is said in Oriental medicine, to stimulate the 'Wei Ch'i' or defensive energy, a Chinese term for what we would call the immunity. Studies at the University of Texas's MD Anderson Hospital found that in cancer patients the activity of T-cells, white blood cells which are a cornerstone of the immunity, were only one third normal. However if cancer patients took extract of astragalus root their T-cells became even more active than in healthy people. Experiments with laboratory animals show that astragalus can prevent the spread of cancer during treatment. At the Cancer Institute in Peking these herbs were given to patients with advanced liver and lung cancer, along with radiation and chemotherapy. The herbs protected the functions of the glands, improved the production of blood, and increased survival from 30 per cent to 70 per cent over one year.

Astragalus and ligusticum have been investigated at the National Cancer Institute and at other centres in the US and found to restore the immune system in 90 per cent of cancer patients. These herbs should be taken on the advice of a herbalist who will also be able to obtain them for you as they are not yet sold widely in Europe. They are more readily available, however, in the US. Your local traditional acupuncturist or Oriental medical practitioner will also be able to locate a source. The dose should be five to ten grams per day of the herbs, taken in combination.

Soviet scientists have also found that eleutherococcus, 'Siberian ginseng' can prevent the biological stress of surgery which would otherwise result in spreading of the cancer. One example among a multitude of Soviet studies was carried out at the Petrov Oncological Institute in Leningrad. There, five grams of eleutherococcus or a look-alike placebo were given every day to 107 patients receiving surgery and chemotherapy for stomach cancer, and the herb or placebo were continued for a year afterwards. Patients given the eleutherococcus were able to tolerate 50 per cent more anticancer drugs, they felt better during treatment, and their average lifespan was increased. These studies have resulted in the Soviets using eleutherococcus widely to improve the resistance of patients to cancer treatment. Both eleutherococcus and ginseng are not so strongly immune-stimulating as the Chinese plants discussed in the previous paragraph, but they do have additional benefits to general vitality, energy and the sense of well-being. The doses are in the region of five grams per day.

Ginseng is well known for its ability to help cope with stress. This includes the debility produced by chemotherapy and radiotherapy. Professor Brekhman of the USSR Academy of Sciences, the father figure of research into the Oriental 'adaptogenic' remedies, found that animals lived twice as long after radiation when they were given ginseng or eleutherococcus. During the last few years a team of scientists led by Dr Yonezawa of Osaka Prefecture Radiation Centre have investigated how ginseng does this, concluding that it is because it gives a sharp boost to the blood factories of the body. I have had several reports from people who described how ginseng has helped them with tiredness, illness and debility during cancer treatment, and for these purposes ginseng appears to be uniquely effective. For advice on taking ginseng see Chapter 3.

The immune-stimulating mushrooms, in particular Ganoderma and Reishi, are being increasingly used by naturopaths as support for patients receiving chemotherapy and radiotherapy. There has been significant research on these therapeutic mushrooms in China, Japan and Russia. For example at the All-Union Cancer Research Center of the USSR Academy of Medical Sciences in Moscow, the late Dr Vladimir Kupin headed a special laboratory to look at how immune-supporting herbs could help cancer patients. The 'Laboratory of Biological Modifiers of Antitumor Immunity' has published over many years a stream of clinical studies demonstrating how eleutherococcus and other Eastern herbs were able to restore white blood cell function, interferon levels and general health and resistance. However they recently came across Ganoderma, and in their opinion it is the best of all immune supporting remedies.

Acupuncture can have similar effects to Chinese herbs but this depends very much on the acupuncturist. He should be a top class *traditional* acupuncturist, who has had experience of looking after cancer patients. If possible, your acupuncturist ought to have a familiarity with Oriental herbs to be able to provide you with the necessary herb combinations. A young research chemist with Hodgkins disease told us that:

'I had chemotherapy two weeks in every month for six months, and acupuncture after each two-week period. After chemotherapy treatment I would always plummet right down; acupuncture did delay plummeting but did not avoid it totally...now feel that I should have had it straight after the injections and it might have helped more...after radiotherapy I felt totally washed out. I had no strength or energy and could hardly get out of a chair...Acupuncture was the only treatment that kept me going. It gave me energy and I could get around.'

There are immune-stimulating herbs in European tradition, but they do not appear to be as strong or well-tried as the Chinese herbs. However one plant, mistletoe (*Viscum album*), has long been used for cancer treatment in Europe. The plant has similar starch-like substances to some of the Oriental remedies described above, and acts as an immune stimulant. For this reason its use just before and during conventional cancer treatments can help prevent spreading of the cancer. In several hospital studies mistletoe preparations have increased survival well above predictions, and it has helped patients to recover energy, health and appetite. Like the other remedies it should be used with the advice of a herbalist.

Chapter Six

DEALING WITH DRUGS AND THEIR SIDE EFFECTS

Why side effects?

Modern drugs began to be made in the middle of the last century by chemists. They took some of the common herbs into the laboratory and out came chemicals which did spectacular things to symptoms. For example aspirin, from witch hazel, made fevers plummet, digoxin, from foxglove, kept hearts pumping regularly. The public rushed to welcome the new miracle remedies. The herbalists at the time made an anguished complaint that these chemicals were strong and harmful, and they treated only the symptoms leaving the disease itself to fester. Voltaire accused physicians of prescribing 'medicines of which they know little, to cure diseases of which they know less in human beings of which they know nothing.'

Despite the incredible sophistication of modern research, the same problems remain today. Chemicals are picked out as drugs because they have obvious effects on laboratory animals. That means that only the strong ones, that really make a rat's whiskers twitch, are selected. Side effects are to be expected. They are natural effects of strong drugs that happen to be the ones we don't want. Safety checking is always partial. For example drugs cannot be tested on human babies.

Codeine, for example, is used to stop coughing, which it does. But as it has a strong action against symptoms, it keeps mucus in the lungs and causes constipation, tiredness and stress on the liver. It actually slows recovery from the disease. These are mild side effects. Sulfonamides, the precursors of modern antibiotics were widely used to protect normal premature babies in hospital from infections, until it was realised that they caused brain damage. Thalidomide was an apparently harmless sedative. Millions of people took and still take the apparently harmless bacteria-killing drug clioquinol ('Enterovioform') for holiday stomach upsets. Yet thousands of Japanese became permanently disabled after the drug ate away their nerves.

The drastic side effects caused by such drugs would be more understandable if the drugs were a vital contribution to health, that is, we know there is no alternative and the risks have been explained. No one is going to sue a drug company for loss of hair during chemotherapy. But much of the side effect problem is the result of drugs which are more or less unnecessary. In the above examples coughs, a good night's sleep, holiday tummy and the vulnerability of premature babies (see Chapter 8) are all treatable by safe, natural methods.

All drugs are poisons to a greater or lesser extent. But whether or not you will get a noticeable side effect depends on dosage, the health of the body's waste-disposal systems in the kidney and liver, constitution, general health and resistance, age, diet, and many other factors. Doctors can never predict who will get which side effect. It is also a question of sensitivity. A healthy person may feel a side effect which is not felt by his unhealthy cousin. It may be that he is more aware of what's going on inside. Even if drug side effects don't produce clear symptoms, it doesn't mean that they are not there. They may only appear later, as with antibiotics. Or they may appear when the dose is raised or when an additional drug is taken. For example tinnitus, ringing in the ear, is a very common and mild side effect. In the US 36 million people have it, often from barbiturates and diuretics. It tends to turn up when tobacco, alcohol or coffee are taken as well as the medical drug.

One in two adults take a drug every day, and children, when ill, take on average one every day. Doctors have 4000 drugs to choose from and fill seven prescriptions per person per year in the UK and more in the US. Given the power of drugs, no wonder side effects are so prevalent. The massive Boston Collaborative Drug Survey checked nearly 25,000 people who were prescribed drugs and found one third with side effects. The most common were from tranquilizers, sedatives, antibiotics, diuretics, painkillers, heart drugs, steroids and anti-inflammatory drugs. Total cost of dealing with side effects in the US...$3 billion.

Your doctor should be on the lookout for bad reactions to drugs. Unfortunately it is not always easy to distinguish drug reactions from symptoms of the disease or a new disease. For example patients who had severe side effects to their eyes and intestinal organs from the blood pressure lowering drug Practolol were for years being given more drugs against supposed neuroses, anxiety, migraines, multiple sclerosis, until the truth eventually dawned on their doctors.

If a side effect occurs the doctor will often replace the drug with a similar one, or change the dosage. Occasionally other drugs can be given to help overcome side effects such as dizziness, nausea, or inflammation, or whatever symptom may turn up. This piling of drug on drug invariably worsens general health. Clearly doctors' options are limited by the fact that for 150 years they have only had sledgehammers with which to crack nuts.

How to avoid drug side effects

The best guards against drug side effects are the doctor's good prescribing habits, your watchfulness and awareness and an understanding between the two of you that drugs should not be a first resort. This requires that your doctor is not conditioned to reach for the prescription pad when he sees you. Choosing such a doctor is discussed in Chapter 2. Suffice to say here that old habits die hard, and often older doctors may be more likely to prescribe excessively than young doctors. You must make it very clear that you don't like to take drugs. 90 per cent of the drugs prescribed in the modern world are not for proper diseases. You don't need them.

Ask your doctor whether the drug really is necessary. Will the problem go away by itself anyway? Is it trivial? Ask yourself: Are you going to the doctor automatically? Is a drug actually what you need? If you feel the weight of modern life will a tranquilizer really lift it, or will it make you more helpless? Is it better to eat more salads and greens for life or be on laxatives for life? Are the blood pressure drugs worth it or is it better to try and change a few habits?

Try preventive methods of treating common problems before exploring the drug option. Many frequent symptoms such as tension-headache, sore throat, frequent colds and infections, digestive upsets, skin irritations, anxiety, mild depression or circulatory problems in their early stages, are very successfully treated by a change in diet, more exercise and fresh air, reducing the pollution inside your body, taking a good break, relaxation and massage. Alternative and holistic medicine is another option. Alternative medical professionals can help you to create the conditions for health so that you will have no need of any drugs.

If a drug is necessary then remember that your doctor should have a *clear aim in mind* when prescribing. Then he should be able to assess if the target has been reached. You can help by asking why the drug is chosen, whether it is to treat the disease or only a symptom, if the symptom, for how long, and what to do then. You should ask what to do if there is no benefit and what problems may arise. Ask about the latest research on this drug.

Your ten questions

1 What is the drug called? What type of drug is it? (The first gives you the brand name, e.g. 'Achromycin', the second question should give you the generic name e.g. tetracycline.)
2 What does the drug do?
3 Why do I need it? Do you know of any non-drug options for treatment?
4 What will happen if I don't take it? Will the problem clear up anyway?
5 Will I be able to stop taking it easily?
6 When and how should I take it?
7 What are the possible side effects? What might happen?
8 How long should I take it for and when should I see results?
9 Are there any foods, drinks, supplements or medicines I shouldn't take?
10 When do you want to see me again?

The eleventh question is one often forgotten, and it could be the most important:

11   May I stop the other drugs I am already taking?

Be wary of any unfamiliar new drug, if an older well-established one is available. When you hear: 'I want to try something new', ask what's wrong with the old.

When you buy and take drugs...

- Never assume that a drug is harmless and it won't hurt to try it. A completely harmless drug is yet to be invented.
- Never assume that if a little works then more will work better.
- A mixture of ingredients is not necessarily better than a single one and may be more toxic.
- When you buy a drug over-the-counter (OTC) at the pharmacy make sure you know the answers to the ten questions. If not, ask the pharmacist.
- Keep to the doctor's or pharmacist's instructions on how to take your drug. If he says take it with meals three times a day, do just that: it will minimize harmful effects.
- If you are in doubt take a drug with food rather than without.
- Don't use old drugs. They may have lost their value and some, such as tetracyclines, can be more harmful when old.

Watching for drug side effects

You need to be on the lookout for unwanted effects. You cannot leave that to your doctor. Be aware of any changes in symptoms, or feelings, even subtle ones like irritability, dryness in your mouth, itching, or tiredness. They may be signs that something is not going well – the tip of the iceberg of invisible damage being created in your body.

A very useful tool for watching what's going on is a diary. Make a daily note of how you feel and whether your original problem is disappearing or new ones are appearing. Sometimes the months pass, and you may just get used to being ill, without realizing that you are now suffering from drug effects different from your original problem.

On page 159 there is a check-list of symptoms that are frequently produced by drugs. It may help you to focus accurately on anything that crops up.

How to know more

Your doctor may not tell you what you want to know; perhaps he doesn't know himself. It may be that the doctor doesn't believe that you have side effects, or doesn't understand how you feel. He is often so influenced by drug companies' advertisements that he believes them rather than you. In such cases you may need independent information.

The classical medical sources of information are the *Physicians Desk Reference* (PDR) in the US and the *British National Formulary* (BNF) in the UK. These are available in libraries and your doctor will have the most recent edition. Look up the drug by name and category. Check the contra-indications (health situations in which the drug must not be given) and its adverse effects.

Another source of information is the *drug datasheet*, a summary of information about the drug compiled by the manufacturer and sent to all doctors who will have it on file. Ask to look at it. If your doctor resists, there are strategies to obtain more information discussed in Chapter 2. The best one is: 'You must accept that a co-operative patient has the best chance of getting better. But how do you expect me to be co-operative without being fully informed?'

A third source is the leaflet in your medicine's packaging. Such leaflets are placed in all packets of over-the-counter (OTC) drugs, but not with prescription drugs. However you can ask the pharmacist to show it to you. Many authorities argue strongly for information leaflets to be given automatically to all patients, however this is not yet done.

All the above sources are in medical language. You may need a

Do you have any of these symptoms while taking drugs?

Affected part	Symptom	Affected part	Symptom
Eyes	Double vision Watering Blurred vision Yellowing of whites Dryness	Muscles	Muscle pain esp. neck Muscle cramps Muscle weakness Tremors/shakes Numbness
Ears and nose	Ringing in ears Pain in ears Bad smells/tastes	Digestion	Dry mouth or thirst Loss of appetite
Skin	Itch or rash Sun sensitivity Flushing Yellowing Unusual sweating Feeling of insects crawling		Diarrhoea or constipation Heartburn Nausea/vomiting Stomach pain or cramps Bloody or black stools
Mind and head	Irritability Dizziness Fainting Frequent yawning Apathy and lethargy Unsteadiness/ lightheadedness Headaches Depression Lack of concentration Insomnia Loss of memory Panic Hallucinations Hyperactivity	Urine	Incontinence Painful or frequent urination Cloudy or dark urine
		General	Unexpected fevers Chills Puffiness, esp. hands, feet Swelling Unexpected weight loss or gain Unusual menstruation or heavy bleeding Loss of sexual drive Impotence
Chest and throat	Constricted throat Breathlessness Unusually rapid or slow heartbeat Chest pain Palpitations		

dictionary. Popular guides include Peter Parish's *Medicine: A Guide For Everybody* (Penguin); L. Gerlis's *Consumer's Guide to Prescription Medicines*; Harold Silverman's *The Pill Book: Guide to Safe Drug Use.*

Incidentally, it will help you to know how drugs are named. Each drug is given a *brand name* by the company (for instance, 'Penbritin' in the UK or 'Omnipen' in the US). Various brands may actually be the same chemical, dressed up in different clothes. Sometimes there will be no brand name, and it will be labelled only by the chemical name. The name of the chemical is the *generic name* (for instance, ampicillin). The actual chemical will belong to a group of chemicals of the same *chemical type* (for instance, penicillins). Various chemical types are classified according to *the purpose* for which they are used (for instance, antibiotic). The diagram below illustrates this example. To know your drug you need to know the purpose, the generic name and the brand name.

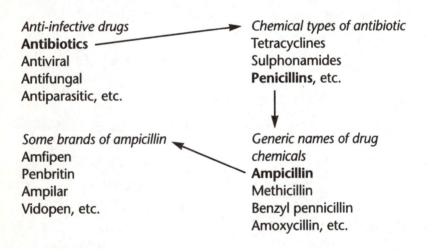

Anti-infective drugs	*Chemical types of antibiotic*
Antibiotics	Tetracyclines
Antiviral	Sulphonamides
Antifungal	**Penicillins**, etc.
Antiparasitic, etc.	
Some brands of ampicillin	*Generic names of drug chemicals*
Amfipen	
Penbritin	**Ampicillin**
Ampilar	Methicillin
Vidopen, etc.	Benzyl pennicillin
	Amoxycillin, etc.

Stopping medical drugs

People having a bad time with drugs often just stop taking them, without telling their doctors. This is patronizingly called 'non-compliance' by the medical profession – not doing what you are told. Two out of five people do not take their medicines as directed, or at all. This is very often because of side effects. But there are a few things you should know before you throw your drugs out of the window.

Very often the symptoms that made you take the drugs in the first place will hit you twice as hard when you stop them. Therefore you should be prepared to put something in their place, either alternative medicine, self-care or a complete break in your usual routine. For example stopping laxatives may bring on greater constipation than before, requiring a thorough dietary change. Stopping decongestants and nasal sprays may make your nasal passages more stuffed up than they were before, and you may need to go to a homoeopath or herbalist for relief.

In the case of some drugs the suppressed symptoms return with such force that you put yourself at real risk if you stop suddenly. This is the case with drugs for the circulation, psychiatric and mood-altering drugs, muscle-relaxants, anti-epileptic drugs and, particularly, steroids. There are also cases, especially antibiotics or anticancer drugs, where withdrawal in mid-course can worsen the disease. Your doctor will be able to advise you on any risks of stopping the drugs. Where there are risks the drugs should be tailed off gradually with the help of a alternative therapist or holistic practitioner who can substitute safer treatment bit by bit. This is discussed more fully below. Where there is no risk, you can indeed throw them away. But don't retrieve them again from the rubbish bin; don't take drugs in a chaotic off-on way. You are safer taking drugs properly or not at all.

Which vitamins should I take to help prevent drug side effects?

A good deal of knowledge has now been gathered on the inter-connections between drugs and dietary factors. Many drugs remove vitamins from the body by using them up, or by preventing their absorption in the digestion from food you eat, or by killing bacteria in the intestine on which you depend. Some drug side effects may result. For example barbiturates put a load on the liver and disturb the machinery there which gets vitamin D ready for the bones. So taking vitamin D along with sleeping pills will prevent bone weakness. Many drugs gradually weaken the kidney leading to a profound lack of vitality and general health. This deterioration can be partly prevented by a diet rich in potassium, magnesium and vitamin B6. Cases of tiredness, loss of memory, confusion and irritation that arise from drugs can sometimes be relieved by B vitamins. It is always helpful to take antioxidant herbs when there is above average level of internal pollution. So you can also take vitamin E and C in normal doses during this time.

Some drugs remove minerals, either because the drugs affect the kidney, making it a leaky sieve (for instance, diuretics), or because they prevent proper absorption from the food (for instance, laxatives), or because the stomach wall is damaged (for instance, neomycin).

The specific vitamin and mineral losses are given in the following tables. (The information is compiled from a number of sources including Dr Daphne Roe, *Drug Induced Nutritional Deficiencies*, Westport, Connecticut; Oversen, *Drugs*, 18, 278–298 (1979); Mindell, E. and Lee, W.H., *Vitamin Robbers*, Keats, New Canaan). Take above the Recommended Daily Allowance, and spread the vitamin dosage throughout the day, roughly in parallel with the drug dosage.

Drugs that deplete vitamins

Type of drug	Purpose of drug	Vitamin depleted
Anticonvulsants, esp. phenytoin	Prevent epileptic seizures	D, K, folic acid, B6
Antacids	Reduce stomach acidity	A, B complex
Aspirin (and salicylates)	Reduce pain, fever, inflammation	A, C, E, K
Barbiturates	Sedatives, sleeping pills	A, D, folic acid, C
Cholestyramine	Lowers cholesterol in blood	A, D, K, folic acid, B complex, B12
Clofibrate	Lowers cholesterol in blood	K
Colchicine	Treats gout	B12, A

Type of drug	Purpose of drug	Vitamin depleted
Corticosteroids	Prevent inflammations and allergies	A, B6, D, C
Diuretics	Increase urination	B complex
Epsom salts	Cleanse the bowels	B2, K
Hydralazine	Lowers blood pressure	B6
Indomethacin	Used in rheumatism and arthritis	B1, C
Isoniazid	Treats tuberculosis	B6, B3
Levodopa	Treats Parkinson's disease	B6
Mineral oil	Laxative	A, D, K
Neomycin	Treats bacterial infections	B12, A
Nitrofurantoin	Treats bacterial infections of the urinary systems	Folic acid
Oestrogen type contraceptives	Contraception (the 'pill')	Folic acid, B6, B12, B2
Penicillamine	Treats rheumatoid arthritis	B6
Phenothiazine	Treats psychosis and schizophrenia	B2
Potassium chloride	Used in potassium deficiency	B12
Pyrimethamine	Prevention and treatment of malaria	Folic acid
Suphasalazine	Treats ulcerative colitis	Folic acid
Tetracycline	Kills bacteria	C
Trimethoprim + sulphonamides	Kills bacteria	Folic acid, K, B

Drugs that deplete minerals

Type of drug	Purpose of drug	Mineral depleted
Anticonvulsants	Prevent epileptic seizures	Calcium
Antacids	Reduce stomach acidity	Phosphate
Aspirin	Reduces pain, fever, inflammation	Iron, phosphate

Type of drug	Purpose of drug	Mineral depleted
Barbiturates	Induce sleeping	Phosphates
Chemotherapeutic drugs	Treat cancerous growth	Magnesium zinc
Colchicine	Treats gout	Sodium, calcium, potassium, iron
Cortisone	Prevents inflammation	Calcium, potassium
Diuretics	Increase urination	Potassium, magnesium, zinc
Laxatives	Reduce constipation	Potassium, calcium
Neomycin	Kills bacteria	Sodium, potassium, calcium, iron

There are also certain rare cases where you should not take vitamins with medication because they counteract it. This is why you should inform your doctor about the vitamins you are taking. Cases include:

Type of drug	Purpose of drug	Vitamin
Anticoagulants	Risk of blood clots	Vit. K or large amounts of leafy vegetables reduce effect
Anti-psychotic drugs	Psychoses	Vit. C can reduce effect
Oestrogen	Contraception (the 'pill')	Vit. C reduces effect
Levodopa	Parkinson's disease	B6 and B complex reduce effect

Type of drug	Purpose of drug	Vitamin
Methotrexate	Leukaemia	Folic acid, B2, can reduce effect
Sulphonamides	Urinary infections	Vit. C can cause kidney stones
Tetracyclines	Infections	Iron, milk, reduce absorption

Dietary methods of coping with drug side effects

The lists in the last section may help you avoid the loss of essential vitamins and minerals. But there is a lot more that foods and supplements can do. They can affect absorption and elimination of drugs, they can prevent damage to organs and other side effects, and they can detoxify the body.

A full stomach will slow down the absorption of most drugs. Drugs will have less effect, but over a longer period. For example, if aspirin is taken with food it takes much longer to have an effect, but food will protect the stomach from attack by aspirin. Some drugs are weaker when taken with food because they become stuck to food components, for example the heart-stimulating drug digoxin on bran, and tetracyclines on milk. Some examples are:

Better absorbed on empty stomach	*Better absorbed on full stomach*
Cephalexin (antibiotic)	Anticoagulants (prevent blood clotting)
Cimetidine (treats stomach ulcers)	Chlorothiazide (increases urination)
Digoxin (stimulates heart beat)	Griseofulvin (treats fungal infections)
Erythromycin (antibiotic)	Nitrofurantoin (treats urinary infections)
Metronidazole (treats amoebic and other infections)	Propanolol (treats hypertension)
Penicillin (antibiotic)	Tranquillizers
Tetracycline (antibiotic)	
Theophylline (relieves bronchitis and asthma)	

Milk is a good medium for taking some drugs as it protects the stomach. But do not take tetracycline with milk. Do not take penicillin and other antibiotics with fruit juices or vitamin C as the acid may break up the drug prematurely.

Drugs are removed by the liver and kidney. Therefore you can prevent side effects by helping the liver and kidney get the drug out after it has done its job. The drug should hit and run. In addition the liver and kidney need special protection to make sure they are not damaged by the chemicals they are forced to dispose of.

The liver has waste disposal systems which 'shred' the body's rubbish – waste products from the metabolism and foreign substances. The waste disposal systems may already be heavily used by alcohol, pollutants, food additives, drugs or pesticides. If the machinery is overloaded waste spills over and may damage the liver itself. Waste also keeps circulating around the body leading to poor health.

Drugs which can damage the liver include paracetamol in high doses, sulphonamides (treat infections), salicylates (relieve pain and inflammation), rifampicin (treats tuberculosis), tetracyclines (antibiotics), cancer chemotherapeutic drugs, halothane-type anaesthetics, isoniazid (treats tuberculosis), phenothiazines (treat psychoses and schizophrenia), many steroids including oral contraceptives, drugs against diabetes and drugs against thyroid problems.

The liver is protected by a low-fat, alcohol-free, additive-free and nutritious diet. In addition some food components, particularly the cabbage family and lemons contain substances that help to prime the pumps in the liver.

Many aromatic and resinous spice plants are helpful to the liver and should not be forgotten in the diet. These include fennel, dill, ginger, cinnamon and chilli pepper. A native doctor once treated a friend of mine for an overdose of sedatives in Lahore, Pakistan. His remedy was nothing more nor less than a bowlful of very hot mango pickle. My friend managed to work his way through it, with much sighing and sweating, and indeed the expected symptoms were prevented.

One of the main housekeeping tools in the liver is a sulphur-containing substance termed glutathione. The antioxidants vitamins C, E and selenium restore glutathione, as does cysteine, one of the natural amino acids. These food factors are the most important of all for helping the liver detoxify drugs, and can protect people who are highly sensitive. For example, French scientists gave one gram of vitamin C and 600 milligrams of vitamin E per day to people who kept getting asthma and skin rashes when they took drugs against arthritis. The side effects were completely abolished compared to other sensitive patients who received placebos.

Garlic, onion and, to a lesser extent, radish and horseradish contain selenium and compounds like cysteine. Garlic has been proved to protect the liver from damage by chemicals.

A healthy kidney is just as important for removal of drugs as the liver. It is even more sensitive to damage by drugs on their way out of the body. Almost every drug can affect the kidney, sometimes irreversibly. The kidney is supported by B vitamins such as B6, and by the best possible environment in the inner sea bathing the tissues of the body. The body water should be made slightly alkaline by alkaline foods particularly vegetables, salads and grains rather than acids such as sugars and starches. Sufficient magnesium and potassium will help the kidney eliminate drugs. These are found in seeds, nuts and green leafy vegetables and salads, preferably organically grown. You should also drink a lot of water and juices to help the kidney filter out the poisons. Vegetable juices would combine all the above requirements. The kidney is also protected by a low-protein diet.

Quite a few drugs are also eliminated by the bile and through the digestion. To help in the elimination of these drugs you need a diet with plenty of roughage, and a helpful normal bacterial zoo in the intestine. This means more plant protein at the expense of animal protein, and as much of a natural wholefood semi-vegetarian diet as possible, with plenty of fruit and yoghurt.

Summarizing, here are some nutritional guidelines to help in drug elimination and to protect your kidneys and liver:

■ Avoid all alcohol, refined oils, animal fats, extra salt, additives, preservatives, chemicals of any kind, smoking and heavy, meaty diets.

- Take one gram of vitamin C, 200 IU vitamin E and 50 milligrams of vitamin B complex (make sure it has B6 as a major component) twice a day.
- Drink vegetable juices and fruit juices plus pure water totaling at least 1.5 litres a day.
- Eat root vegetables, fruit, dark green leafy vegetables especially the cabbage family, salads, alfalfa and other sprouts, garlic and onion. But discuss your diet with your doctor if you are taking anticoagulants.
- Eat lentils, grains, seeds (e.g. sunflower, sesame or pumpkin), soya products, beans, fish and liver.
- Supplemental foods should include yeast, fish liver oil and selenium-containing foods such as garlic or selenium-yeast, and live yoghurt.
- Use unrefined, cold-pressed oil especially sunflower, sesame or olive oil.
- Take specific vitamins or minerals that are removed by the drug concerned (see Table on page 163).

Special protection for the over 60s...

One of the commonest afflictions of the elderly is loss of memory, concentration and clarity. Sometimes this is senile dementia or Alzheimer's disease which is irreversible. But it may often be due to drugs and can be reversed. Only the bravest of doctors used to admit, quietly, that he had cured some of his demented elderly patients by taking them off all drugs. Now the *British Medical Journal* (27/10/1984) stated in a leading article that it is surprising that the elderly who take drugs can pass any mental tests. It advised that drugs should be suspected in all cases of mental deterioration in the elderly, and *any* drug can be to blame.

Elderly people take more drugs because they have more problems, they may have had more years of drug damage, and their liver and kidneys are weaker. Drugs stay around much longer in the blood of older people. It is mostly the elderly who are hospitalized by severe drug side effects. The major culprits are anti-depressants, steroid and non-steroid analgesics, anti-inflammatory or antirheumatic drugs (taken by two out of three elderly people), heart drugs, diuretics, sedatives, antidiabetic drugs, tranquilizers and drugs for incontinence.

It is tempting to keep taking OTC drugs such as antacids, painkillers, and laxatives. But long term use of these drugs can cause all sorts of complications. For example bone and heart problems may arise because the balance of sodium and potassium, and other minerals, has gone haywire. So:

- Ensure that you are getting the right information from your doctors. A US Food and Drug Administration (FDA) survey found that three quarters of the over 60s in the US were not told by their doctor how to take their drugs safely, nor about possible side effects. Make sure you regularly review what drugs you are taking with your doctor, including any over-the-counter drugs, and see if you can dispense with any.
- Try to withdraw from over-the-counter medicines, especially antacids and painkillers. Bulk laxatives such as bran or ispaghula husks are safe; chemical laxatives are not.
- Use daily vitamin supplements and dietary recommendations are described above. Add iron if using painkillers and anti-inflammatory drugs. Add vitamins A, D and folic acid, and vitamin B12, which are the commonest deficiencies in the elderly.
- Take potassium supplements and magnesium-rich food if you are taking diuretics or antacids with bicarbonate, or sodium penicillin, or other sodium-containing drugs.

...And the under 1s

At the other end of the lifespan the very young are also vulnerable because their systems for removing drugs, poisons and waste are still under development. An unborn baby may take several times as long to eliminate the drug as the mother and being so tiny becomes loaded with a drug that hardly makes a difference to the mother. This is discussed in Chapter 8 in relation to drugs given to the mother at birth. However *all drugs* taken during pregnancy are a potential risk and their effects on the unborn and the newborn are largely unknown.

Anticoagulants, the antibiotic chloramphenicol, anticancer agents, the anti-infective sulphonamides, lithium, barbiturates, cholesterol-reducing drugs, anti-inflammatory/antirheumatics, anti-gout drugs, thiazide diuretics, tranquilizers, oral contraceptives, steroids, the anti-infective metranidazole, anti-gastric ulcer drugs, diet pills and appetite suppressants, tetracycline antibiotics, bronchial dilators and the anti-epileptic phenytoin, are all drugs that should be avoided at all costs while pregnant or breast feeding. They go through into the milk.

If possible *avoid all drugs* when pregnant or breast-feeding. You can assume that all drugs affect the baby to some extent, and remember that doctors can't ask the baby how it feels. If a drug is unavoidable, make sure you discuss the risks to your unborn or breast-fed baby. Then watch carefully for any symptoms in the list on page 159. Be alert for unusual behaviour. In any event, try to obtain short-acting drugs which you should take just after breast-feeding, and add the supplements and vitamins discussed. Over-the-counter drugs that affect salt and minerals, such as chemical laxatives, sodium bicarbonate antacids, Epsom Salts, or diuretics can cause problems during pregnancy.

Natural methods of detoxification

After you have stopped taking drugs, symptoms might remain such as tinnitus, tiredness, headaches, skin problems, digestive problems, allergies, or a general feeling of being run-down. They can be helped by detoxification. Long-term use of many drugs can create symptoms which hang on for a year or two afterwards, so detoxification may also take some time. Detoxification is accomplished by several procedures. They should be guided by naturopathic or holistic practitioners.

Partial fasting
Partial fasting should only start after you have stopped the drugs. There are, for example, fruit (grape-juice), raw food, low-calorie,

vegan, and macrobiotic brown rice fasts. An excellent fast is the raw food fast. It is a ten-day fast, in which you eat as much as you want of raw vegetables or sprouts in salad, with a little dressing of cold-pressed oil, wheat germ, yeast and cider vinegar. For two to three days you have nothing else whatsoever. After the third day you add any roasted seeds (but not grains), nuts and more fruit, and after the fifth day you add yoghurt. You only go back to cooked foods and cooked grains after ten days, starting with soups and fish and working slowly up to bread and a full wholefood diet. Drink juices, pure water or herb teas and a daily couple of cups of one to two tablespoons of cider vinegar in hot water with honey to taste.

Do not take vitamin supplements during the fast as you need to be cleaned out of all external chemicals, even fillers in vitamin pills. After that time take a continuous daily supplementation of: vitamin C 1000 milligrams, vitamin E 200 IU, vitamin A 10,000 units and B complex 100 milligrams.

Exercise and sauna baths
Exercise regularly every day. As it says in the Vedic books, it should bring at least three drops of sweat to your brow! Sweating is an important cleansing process and removes drug wastes. Doing it through exercise is more beneficial to the organs than using a sauna. Exercise such as swimming, skiing, football, rowing, running, aerobic dancing etc., are all good. Practice deep breathing as you exercise. But always start exercising gradually. After exercise have a thorough wash, and scrub the skin of your back, torso and stomach. Exercise is an excellent cure for bouts of depression, fatigue or temptation to take further unnecessary drugs or toxins.

Saunas are useful but only when you have stopped taking the medical drugs. You should not take saunas or sudden vigorous exercise along with several kinds of drugs, which are, incidentally, also more dangerous in a hot climate. They include antihistamines, beta-blockers and other high blood pressure drugs, antidepressants, amphetamines, diuretics, anticoagulants and phenothiazines. Ask your doctor about vigorous exercise and heat if you take these drugs.

Health farms
It is worth considering health farms or special detoxification centres if you can afford them. They can help to complete the process much more quickly. Some of the tricks of the trade are:

■ Coolish saunas for two hours every day.
■ Several spoons of vegetable oil a day to mobilize body fat, vitamin supplementation including high doses of B3 and other B vitamins, and antioxidants.
■ Exercise programmes under supervision.
■ Hydrotherapy.
■ Herbal teas and tisanes to aid elimination and purification.

Herbs for detoxification
These include bitter-aromatic herbs, which stimulate the function of the liver. These can be very effective in removing toxins which are eliminated by an extra flow of bile. The herbs include wormwood, angelica root, myrrh and gentian. They should be combined with herbs that purify the blood and help the liver protect and repair its waste-disposal systems. Chief herb here is milk-thistle. The active component, silymarin, has been found to have a truly amazing ability to treat liver poisoning and hepatitis. Others are globe artichoke extract, dandelion root, agrimony and turmeric.

At the same time the kidneys should be helped to eliminate the toxins. Mild diuretics include nettle, parsley seed or carrot seed. Parsley, nettle, dandelion or alfalfa leaves, kelp and radish are excellent to restore the right balance of minerals in the body, improve absorption and elimination, increase vigor and energy and improve sleep. Unlike the other herbs these can be taken without the need for a visit to a herbalist, at a total dose of 25 grams of dried leaf daily, or the equivalent quantity of fresh leaf, or tincture.

Acupuncture
Acupuncture can be very useful for restoring kidney and liver function. Moreover acupuncture is able to make you feel better, lighter and more purposeful, and therefore more able to continue with a self-help detoxification programme. When 20,000 Japanese received partial paralysis as a side effect of the stomach remedy

clioquinol (in Enterovioform), the Japanese government provided them with the means to obtain acupuncture and herbal treatment to speed their return to health.

Homoeopathic 'scrubs'
These are the homoeopathic version of blood purifying and eliminative remedies. Typical remedies include nux vomica (×6) with sulphur (×6) or with pulsatilla (×6) depending on the individual constitution. They should be used to remove toxins as part of an overall homoeopathic treatment.

Alternative medicine and drug side effects

It would be wonderful if you could go to the doctor for a drug to cure a disease and go to a herbalist to mop up all the side effects. The best of both worlds. Actually it doesn't work that way. Modern drugs tend to deal with symptoms not cures, and if you go to a herbalist for advice on drug side effects he may surprise you by attempting to cure the disease. This does not mean that he can do nothing about drug induced suffering. It is that his aim will always be to take you off the drugs altogether.

For example a woman in her early 30s went to a herbalist complaining of thrush, a fungal infection in the genital area, while on a long chain of courses of antibiotics for a bladder infection. The thrush is a clear side effect of the antibiotics. The herbalist helped with garlic pills and a cider-vinegar douche. At the same time he prevented the antibiotics from doing further damage by prescribing Lactobacillus acidophilus tablets and live yoghurt three times a day. This was combined with a strict dietary regime, together with St John's wort and other herbs to clear out the infection. The woman came off antibiotics permanently at the end of the course she was taking.

Drug side effects create problems for alternative practitioners because they muddy the waters. They suppress the symptom picture of the disease and substitute symptoms of their own. For example alternative medicine would under normal circumstances treat rheumatic problems by working on the circulation and the liver to alter the metabolism which creates deposits in the joints.

But anti-inflammatory drugs create liver, kidney and digestive system damage which are superimposed on, and hide, the original liver problem. 'The drugs,' said one practitioner, 'come between me and the patient.' Steroids are a very serious problem in this respect, and homoeopaths especially find that they create such a weird, alien internal world in the body of the patient that the homoeopathic approach hardly works.

Nevertheless it is the alternative practitioner's job to disentangle all this, and he may do it in a number of ways. He may just treat whichever is bothering the patient most, the disease or the side effects. Or he may treat both at once. If the drugs are addictive, such as painkillers, tranquilizers, steroids and anti-inflammatory drugs, he may support the patient by gentle remedies which gradually replace the drugs. Then, when the patient is off the drugs and the original condition is exposed or flares up, it can be treated. The path is flexible. No two people will be treated by the same formulae. This whole process takes time. A rule of thumb estimate is a month of treatment for every year of the disease. But the goal of a holistic treatment is a *complete* cure.

Alternative practitioners see a great variety of drug side effect problems. Indeed many will say that they are frustrated by constantly having to deal with doctor-caused ill-health rather than the root of the health problems. Some of the main drug side effects which constantly turn up in practitioners clinics, and how they deal with them, are described in the following chapter. It deals with specific categories of drugs and what we can do about them.

'Hair-of-the-dog'

Homoeopaths select their remedies according to the principle of 'Like-Cures-Like'. The remedy that creates certain symptoms in a healthy person will negate those same symptoms in the sick. If a set of symptoms, such as spasm and diarrhoea during dysentery, are like those produced by a certain poison, e.g. arsenic, then arsenic (in infinitesimal dosage) can be used as a cure.

One discovery, made by both European and Indian homoeopaths, is that very small doses of drugs or any poisons will help the body to eliminate the same poison. This is like using fire to fight fire. The method, called *isopathic* homoeopathy, is simple. To eliminate a drug from the body and help deal with its side effects, the homoeopath would heavily dilute a little of the drug in a special way ('potentization') and give it to the patient in drops or pills. For example a patient came to a London homoeopath after receiving the highly toxic drug isotretinoin ('Roaccutane'in UK, 'Accutane' in US) against acne. The drug had cleared up the acne but just as the acne disappeared side effects appeared – an intense burning in the chest, and all the sweat glands shut down. The young man couldn't wash and couldn't sleep. He was given an antidote made of a high homoeopathic dilution of the drug plus basic constitutional remedies to work on the cause of the original acne. Gradually both the basic problem and the side effects cleared up.

Homoeopaths in the UK vary in their attitude to isopathy. Some say that such antidoting is bad for the patient in the long run as it further obscures the original condition. Others will use antidotes of tranquilizers, antibiotics, steroids and other drugs to help patients overcome their dependencies, always along with more conventional homoeopathic treatment. It has not yet been fully evaluated homoeopathically. Of course as far as conventional medicine is concerned, isopathy is still in the realms of wizardry.

Herbal self-help for specific drug side effects

Herbs can treat certain drug-induced symptoms. But as long as you continue to take the drug which creates them, it is like baling a leaky boat. Nevertheless there will be cases where herbs are so needed to relieve drug induced suffering that even in a second-best role of assistant to drug treatment they are valuable. Here are some self-help suggestions. They should not replace determined action to obtain real healing.

Stomach pains and cramps
One or two drops of peppermint oil or hot peppermint tea several times a day; pains after food can be relieved by the digestive enzymes bromelain (or pineapple juice) and pepsin (or a fresh papaya), and by making tea from, or chewing, fennel, caraway or

aniseed. Pain from drug attacks on the stomach lining can be helped by slippery elm, liquorice root, Icelandic moss and alginates or seaweed products.

Loss of appetite
Aromatic bitters, especially sweet flag, angelica and gentian, taken as a few drops of tincture in water before meals; alfalfa and 50 to 100 milligrams of B complex taken with meals may help to stimulate appetite.

Nausea and vomiting
Chew a teaspoonful of fresh ginger, or add one gram of dried ginger to a herb tea. Strong chamomile tea can also help. If nausea is combined with gas use aniseed or fennel seeds, chewed or as teas, as well.

Constipation
Alder buckthorn, crushed linseed, and aloes are helpful. Enrich the diet with bran, ground linseed or ispaghula husks together with mucilaginous foods like prune juice or figs. Stronger laxatives include senna and cascara. Drink a lot.

Diarrhoea
Live yoghurt, especially taken with ispaghula husks, helps. Try slippery elm (put 25 grams in 1.1 litres of water and bring to the boil), or cooked blueberries and blackberries and a tea from blackberry root bark or raspberry leaf; enrich the diet with bananas, carob flour and barley.

Insomnia
Teas (or products) of hops and valerian or a strong chamomile tea before bedtime help, along with outdoor exercise during the day. Vitamin B6 before bedtime can be useful.

Anxiety/nervousness
Herb teas or tinctures of balm, valerian or passiflora, combined with hawthorn if there are palpitations, will reduce these symptoms. Progressive relaxation or hypnosis are very effective.

Skin rashes and dermatitis

Heartsease or golden seal tea externally and once a day internally; use extra vitamin E and C with bioflavonoids in the diet; vitamin E in wheat germ oil helps itching. Quercitin is a potent anti-histamine and antioxidant flavonoid substance originally found in oak, but known in many other herbs. It is very effective at stopping rashes and eczema. It can now be bought in capsules for internal use. Also use calendula, oak bark or strong chamomile tea applied as moist compresses to treat eczema.

Headache

Rosemary and fresh ginger tea, willow bark tablets, lavender oil or rue for smelling, peppermint tea and mentholated balms applied to forehead and nape of neck can help, followed by warmth (especially of hands and feet) and relaxation/meditation. Learn the acupressure points for headaches. Headache may often be the result of liver problems which should be treated as on page 166.

Tiredness

Try supplementing your diet with B vitamins and one gram of vitamin C. Herbal tonics include ginseng with a spare nutritious diet and exercise in the fresh air. Kola nut and damiana may help. Smell basil oil, and add a few drops to your bath.

Cold hands and feet

Rosemary tea or oil or cinnamon oil (two drops internally) and exercise; also deep relaxation. Use cramp bark, angelica, ginger and lobelia in a tea mixture. Massage with rosemary or mustard oil.

Tinnitus

Treat nutritionally by excellent diet and multivitamins, especially A and C. Deep relaxation helps. Take summer savory tea and a drop of the oil in the ear. Balm and valerian tea may also help.

In the above cases, the average dose for tea would be two to three spoonfuls of dried herbs in a cup of boiling water. You can sometimes also find capsules, or obtain tinctures from a practitioner.

Chapter Seven

RESCUE FROM COMMON DRUGS

Part 1: Drugs affecting the mind: tranquilizers, antidepressants, antipsychotics

Tranquilizers and tranquilizing sedatives

Tranquilizers were originally developed to deal with disabling, nail-chewing anxiety, and anxiety connected with medical procedures, for example before operations. They all belong to the chemical class of *benzodiazepines*. These include diazepam (for instance, 'Valium'), chlordiazepoxide (for instance, 'Librium'), clorazepate (for instance, 'Tranxene'), lorazepam (for instance, 'Ativan') and prazepam ('Centrax'). Other benzodiazepines such as temazepam (for instance, 'Normison' in the UK), flurazepam (for instance, 'Dalmane') and nitrazepam (for instance, 'Mogadon' in the UK) were promoted as sleeping pills, 'safer' alternatives to barbiturates.

Doctors cannot help using tranquilizers as an anodyne for every unspecific pain, grumble or worry that patients bring to the surgery. They have six minutes per patient and tranquilizers are, from their point of view, the perfect complaint stopper. Up to ten out of every 100 people will be taking tranquilizers at any one time. Although the UK's Committee on Safety of Medicines recommended that they shouldn't be used for more than four weeks since the effects wear off after this time, a 1985 MORI poll found that three and a half million people in the UK have taken tranquilizers for more than four months. Two out of ten elderly Americans have used them for more than a year. Most of these people were handed out repeat prescriptions and were not told about side effects or the risk of addiction.

Yet the side effects can include the same problems that the drugs were meant to treat – depression, anxiety, rage, fear, insomnia, suicidal tendencies, and loss of sexual potency, as well as drowsiness, loss of memory, confusion (leading to falls), brain damage and problems with the baby if taken during breast-feeding. Tranquilizers are addictive, even with therapeutic doses. The US Health Research Group reckons that the majority of those taking tranquilizers beyond two months will be addicted. 2000 former tranquilizer addicts sued two drug companies for not telling people how addictive the drugs were.

I had started taking Valium for a back problem beginning with four milligrams a day writes Barbara Gordon in her book on tranquilizer addiction (*I'm Dancing as Fast as I Can*); *Now I was up to 30 milligrams and couldn't get out of the house without taking them.* Her doctor told her they were not addictive. But when she stopped taking them she suffered from a complete mental and physical collapse. The most common withdrawal symptoms are: sleep disturbance, anxiety, pains, tremor, headache, nausea, sweating, visual disturbance, fatigue, hypersensitivity, depersonalization, psychosis and convulsions. The tranquilizers protect people from their emotions and when they are withdrawn the shell is broken '…standing at the bus stop and someone shouts at you, you feel as if you have been punched in the stomach,' is how one young man described it.

If you are taking tranquilizers, please consider two points. First, that they are now known to be no more effective than counselling and may give you new symptoms in the bargain. Secondly, that symptoms of withdrawal may feel like those of the original problem, so you may rush back to the drug assuming you really need it.

If you ask your doctor to withdraw you from the drug he ought to step down the dosage by one eighth every two to four weeks to reach the lowest dose. He may also use different tranquilizers. Another drug, flumazenil ('Anexate' in the UK only), made, ironically, by one of the tranquilizer companies can be used to help withdrawal. However the best medical aid to withdrawal appears to be nicotinic acid (vitamin B3), given in high doses of one to two grams. Ask your doctor or practitioner to check this out, but don't try such high doses of B3 yourself.

Holistic practitioners are likely to help you off tranquilizers in a more delicate and yet thorough way. They would always recommend improved nutrition, presuming that most people who are on tranquilizers wouldn't have been dancing in the kitchen preparing fresh and wholesome meals. The same goes for exercise and breathing. They might teach abdominal breathing or aerobics. Both extra nutrients and proper breathing go a long way to restoring natural positive vitality and countering the symptoms of withdrawal.

Herbal treatment soothes tensions in both mind and body, and relieves withdrawal symptoms. One strategy uses the herbal tranquilizers skullcap and valerian as main herbs, perhaps together with the sedative hops. These gradually replace the chemical tranquilizers. At the same time oat tea may be used to strengthen the nerves, passiflora to prevent palpitations and reduce agitation or tremors, motherwort to support the circulation, and pulsatilla or pasque flower to help with nervous exhaustion. Ginseng will reduce stress and restore basic vitality and 'life-force'. The precise treatment programme must be defined on an individual basis. Some recommend two to four days on drugs plus herbs, then dropping one sixth of the drug dosage every four to five days. Others take the withdrawal much more easily, spreading it over months, shaving off more and more of the pills all the time with a nail file!

Counselling and constant reassurance are an essential part of the treatment. The emotional anaesthesia created by tranquilizers leads to hopelessness and emptiness on withdrawal. Warm, supportive connections between you and a practitioner or friend can make the withdrawal much faster. Massage, especially with essential oils, such as basil or cinnamon, also help to lift mood and bring back self-confidence.

Acupuncture can gradually improve mental and physical health to the point where tranquilizers are about as unnecessary as earplugs at a harpsichord recital. An acupuncturist told us about a 40-year-old man who suffered from a childhood deformity which gave him a permanent limp. At 21 he had had a nervous break-down when someone stole his brand-new car while he was at work, and had been taking medication on and off since then. He had been taking lorazepam ('Ativan') morning and evening for the last seven years and if he forgot one dose he would get immediate panic attacks and vertigo. He came to the acupuncturist with chest pains which were clearly psychological. The acupuncturist treated him regularly and the pains soon receded. After six months he stopped taking Ativan completely and found the will and energy to begin exercise classes, to change his job and start to reevaluate his life.

Antidepressants

We are concerned here with the two main types, the tricyclics such as amitriptyline (for instance, 'Tryptizol' in the UK and 'Elavil' in the US), doxepin (for instance, 'Sinequan'), butriptyline (for instance, 'Evadyne' in the UK), imipramine (for instance, 'Tofranil') and others, or monoamine-oxidase inhibitors (MAOIs) such as tranylcypromine (for instance, 'Parnate'), phenelzine (for instance, 'Nordil').

Antidepressants are not so addictive as tranquilizers but they do have side effects including dizziness, tiredness, dry mouth, blurred vision, headache, constipation, urinary retention, sweating and heart rhythm disturbances. Cases of sudden death of people with weak hearts can occur because of these drugs. They can also lead to impotence and obesity. In a recent study of 93 outpatients given these drugs, 31 per cent started to eat excessively and became obese, and 34 per cent had a craving for sugar. If you stop taking them abruptly the depression returns with interest, or there are other symptoms, so carefully planned withdrawal is necessary.

The main problem is that depression is so poorly understood that antidepressants are vastly over-used. They are given because of a gross oversimplification which sees human suffering as a chemical abnormality in the brain. They only really help those disabled by depression, while most cases are in fact due to psycho-social problems, poor diet and unhealthy lifestyle, low blood pressure and side effects of other drugs. They are also given to children to stop bedwetting, even though this is known to be the result of emotional problems and not helped by drugs.

Those taking antidepressants feel vulnerable because they react with a whole host of other drugs, street drugs such as cocaine, alcohol, and in the case of the older MAOI antidepressants, a range of foods such as cheese, pickles, yoghurt, yeast or chocolate.

Depression can very often be successfully treated by holistic or alternative methods especially where the gloom arises from low vitality. Such methods would include diet, acupuncture, yoga and relaxation, and herbs, which can be combined with counselling or psychotherapy. Diet is surprisingly important, as sugar and carbohydrate-rich refined junk food can make depression worse. This, needless to say, is the kind of food given to patients in mental institutions who take these drugs. The B vitamins, especially B1, B6 and B12, help with depression. They counteract the side effects of antidepressant drugs and the side effects of poor diet. According to some recent research, magnesium and manganese (available in green leafy vegetables, seeds, fish, and some herbs such as nettle) apparently make these drugs safer and more effective, although why is anybody's guess.

There are a number of herbs which can be used as a replacement during and after withdrawal. For example a woman came to see a London herbalist after her doctor had taken her off an amitryptiline antidepressant too fast and she had had a strong reaction. The herbalist gave her a diet which was natural-semivegetarian without coffee and tea. He prescribed kola nut, and damiana as natural mild stimulants, and hyssop and verbena to raise her spirits and bring her successfully through the withdrawal. Ginseng is another herb which is able to assist vitality during the withdrawal period.

If you are taking these drugs, acupuncture can help. It does so by working on the same brain centres that appear to be involved in depression. Besides this, it helps the liver and organs to clean out the drug. It may seem strange that putting needles in your hands can affect your mood and thoughts. However depression is not the result of thoughts, more of the state of mind within which thoughts arrive. It can be viewed as a drain on the flow of life force or, in Chinese terms, the 'ch'i' energy which keeps all bodily activities well adjusted. Acupuncture can alter the rhythms and function of all the organs of the body including the brain. If depression is like a weak and fuzzy picture on the TV, acupuncture is a bit like adjusting it with a screwdriver. Antidepressant drugs are like hitting it with a hammer.

Brian Peters saw a lot of hospitals when he was young. He kept on having accidents and was plagued by headaches and sinus problems. He was very depressed during adolescence and had been given stronger and stronger drugs which he hated, feeling that they were taking his life away. At 18 he was given a combination antidepressant which put him in a state of total panic. He couldn't sleep and felt like a 'crazed junky – wide-eyed and alarmed'. When he tried to stop the drugs every experience became so painful that he soon started them again. He suffered from blinding headaches which mystified migraine clinics, neurosurgeons and hospital doctors but which he eventually found were due to coffee reacting with the drugs. He went on from illness to illness – pancreatitis, orchitis, stomach ulcer, colitis – until he went to a naturopathic osteopath for an injury. This practitioner immediately put him on a strict diet, and prescribed herbal compresses. His positive attitude helped Brian to get better though he kept on getting new health problems. He only fully understood them when he saw an acupuncturist who said that his health had been ruined by liver damage created by the antidepressants. The liver was overworking, or 'burning-up' in acupuncture terms. The acupuncturist drained energy from the liver. When I saw Brian later he was fit as a fiddle, young-looking and energetic.

Antipsychotic drugs

I didn't intend to write about phenothiazine drugs like chlorpromazine ('Largactyl' in the UK, 'Thorazine' in the US), haloperidol (e.g. 'Haldol') and others. These antipsychotic drugs, sometimes misleadingly described as the 'Major Tranquilizers', are only given to psychotic or schizophrenic mental patients. Because of these drugs many people with serious mental problems can lead a worthwhile life within the community. These drugs have emptied the mental homes of psychotics and schizophrenics.

However many people with friends or relatives who were taking these drugs are desperately concerned about the side effects. The scale of the suffering caused by them may not be apparent. Some experts believe they work by brain damage, rather than brain repair. If antidepressants bring a hammer to the TV, the pheno-thiazines rip out some circuits. In 1985 a World Mental Health Congress was shocked to hear that 'More than 25 million patients worldwide have suffered irreversible brain damage as a result of these drugs...four million prescriptions are issued a year in the UK...150 million people worldwide are taking these drugs... Giving people chemicals that cause brain damage to this extent is silly.' This must be the understatement of the year.

The main sign of this brain damage is tardive dyskinesia (t.d.) which is a loss of control over the muscles. It leads to involuntary movements of the tongue and face or jerking and trembling in the body. There are also other quite serious health problems including liver damage, visual disturbances, impotence, and a kind of Parkinson's disease. Doctors are now more expert at planning drug treatment so as to reduce these effects. Nevertheless, because mental patients may be poor at communicating their symptoms, every such patient needs a 'champion' to review their medication continually. These drugs may only be useful in the short term. During the long term they may cause more mental illness than they cure. They should *never* be used simply as sedatives to help 'manage' unstable people. Don't forget that they often substitute for care and attention.

There is little known about how to prevent side effects using alternative medicine. The main effort should be made to limit dosage and the length of time they are taken. Ask the questions listed in Chapter 2 especially: 'Are therapeutic targets clear? For how long are the drugs really necessary?'

Again, a good diet helps to protect organs and minimize damage. Eating should be slow, with small mouthfuls, as it may be harder to cough. Eat a diet rich in magnesium, manganese and zinc, minerals which are important to normal mental function. These can be obtained from greens, nuts and seeds as described elsewhere. Phenothiazines are reported to interfere with riboflavin in the body, so extra vitamin B2 should be taken. The B vitamins can actually be used therapeutically to treat schizophrenia and to prevent t.d. The use of large doses of B vitamin, especially B1 and B3, is described as 'orthomolecular psychiatry'. For example over the last ten years 11,000 patients at the North Nassau Mental Health Center, Manhasset, N.Y. have been given a vitamin formulation with their drugs. Apparently few of them have developed t.d. The formulation consists of capsules containing one third of a gram of vitamin C plus one third of a gram of vitamin B3 plus 66 milligrams of pyridoxine plus 66 IU of vitamin E. Each day four to twelve capsules are taken. These are high doses of the vitamins and should only be taken under supervision of a practitioner.

A new study published in the *American Journal of Psychiatry* has suggested that t.d. is caused by free radicals (see Chapter 2) which attack nerve cells. The study showed that the antioxidant vitamin E could actually treat a majority of the t.d. cases. It would be a wise precaution to take extra vitamin E, up to 1000 I.U. a day, during treatment with these drugs.

Part 2: Antibiotics, steroids, non-steroid anti-inflammatory drugs, blood pressure lowering drugs, OTC painkillers

Antibiotics

The most spectacular results of modern medicine are achieved with antibiotics. They are apparently so successful at killing bacteria and stopping infections that it is virtually heretical to doubt them. And indeed no-one would doubt their value in acute and serious infections that are racing fast.

However most antibiotics are given for pains, inflammation, mild infections or ghosts of infections. Often they are given before a proper diagnosis is made. Studies show that two thirds of the patients in hospital given antibiotics didn't have any signs of bacterial infection. When antibiotics were given routinely to prevent infections, for example in surgery, infections were actually found to be more frequent than if no drugs were given. Infections were caused by tougher bugs or 'super-bugs' which were resistant to the usual antibiotics. One example of the vast over use of antibiotics in the community was pointed out recently in the *British Medical Journal* (14/4/1990). It said that 85 per cent of children with earache don't need antibiotics and nearly two million antibiotic prescriptions given in the UK per year for this problem are useless.

Perhaps worse than useless. For besides the one in 100 that suffer from a severe reaction, antibiotics prevent the body from properly fighting the disease. The body is left with unhealed residues of disease which may cause more serious problems later in life. In addition, antibiotics pull the rug out from under the immune system with the result that the disease is more likely to come back, as most cystitis sufferers understand. Another side effect which is beginning to worry health professionals is that antibiotics don't distinguish friend from foe. They kill off the friendly bacteria which live in and around the body. The intestine has 1.5 kilos of friendly bacteria which help in food absorption, production of vitamins and elimination of poisons. When these are killed new and insidious types take over. This can cause digestive problems (diarrhoea, constipation, nausea, colitis) and build up of poisons in the body (headaches, tiredness, insomnia and so on).

The longer the antibiotics are continued, the more damage is done by the wrong kind of bacteria and yeasts (especially Candida). Holistic physicians are now convinced that allergies and arthritis are common results of long term use of antibiotics.

If you are in good health you should be able to get over virtually all the common infections you are likely to meet, without the need for antibiotics. Antibiotics are an admission of failure of your health care. Good nutrition, exercise, and general self-care while you are healthy will help to see you over most infections without antibiotics. If you do get an infection, don't be afraid of it. If you are confident that most infections will go away by themselves and will not threaten your life you give your immunity a chance to work – that's what it's there for.

I stopped taking medical drugs in 1975 and since then neither my children nor myself have ever had any antibiotics. We do get ill now and then. But if we get a fever, inflammation, sore throat or whatever, we see the symptoms as the expression of the body's defences, and give the immunity a helping hand by fasting, rest-ing, drinking herb teas or using ice-cold compresses for high fever. We also use natural anti-infectives including thyme, sage, hyssop, propolis, echinaceae, yarrow, and, especially, garlic. External infections like boils can be treated by compresses of plantago, golden seal, and tea tree lotion. If the infection stays, or gets worse, over the next few days, or if there are symptoms of a more serious nature (for instance, swollen lymph nodes) we would go to see our family doctor for a diagnosis.

However chronic infections that do not go away can damage health, and should always be treated professionally by a doctor or alternative practitioner. If you go to a doctor concerning an infection, besides the questions suggested in Chapter 2:

■ Check with your doctor if the infection is self-limiting. If so, say that you would prefer to treat it without antibiotics. If it is unusual or progressive you should request the 'mildest' antibiotic, or seek help from a competent herbalist or homoeopath.
■ If your doctor recommends antibiotics ask why he thinks it is a bacterial infection. A laboratory analysis before treatment is often worthwhile to confirm that the antibiotic will actually work. This may help to avoid frequent hit-and-miss over-prescribing.
■ Take the antibiotics, if you have to, for the minimum time (but not less than one full course) and then evaluate from the beginning before accepting a repeat course. If the infection comes back consider going elsewhere.
■ Don't take new fancy antibiotics if the older, more traditional ones will do. Don't take broad spectrum 'scatter-shot' antibiotics if specific ones will do.

If you have to take antibiotics, you can reduce potential side effects by helping to cultivate the normal bacterial garden inside you. Take natural 'live' (especially 'Bulgarian') yoghurt three times a day after the antibiotics. It is best to make the yoghurt yourself at home using a starter culture, so you know it is alive. You can also take tablets of the useful bacteria, Lactobacillus acidophilus or Lactobacillus bulgaricus, and the bifidobacteria, which should be available from a health shop.

Along with Lactobacillus, eat a fibre-rich, low protein diet with plenty of green vegetables, carrots, milk products, fish, eggs and whole grains. There are suggestions that a lot of fruit may encourage yeasts, so eat fruit moderately. Garlic and onion help to remove poisons left by the infection which the body cannot clear out because of the antibiotics. Cayenne pepper will help to distribute and sweat out these toxins. You can kick both the residual antibiotics and the toxins out of the body by detoxification procedures (see page 170) after you have finished the antibiotic course.

As far as supplements are concerned, the most important is half a gram of vitamin C three times a day. You should take extra B vitamins (especially B6 and pantothenic acid) to replace those lost in the intestinal chaos. Manganese (in wheat germ, seeds and the like) can help to prevent the damage to hearing that can occur from neomycin-type drugs. Vitamin E may help to protect the liver and prevent the yellowing of teeth when taking tetracyclines.

If a fungal or yeast infection does occur, it can only be treated by holistic or alternative practitioners, as the conventional antifungal drugs are even worse than most antibiotics. If external (say, thrush), it can be treated by a douche of thyme tea or cider vinegar, and if internal with blood cleansers (thyme, echinaceae, garlic, and so on). If the infection is internal, (for instance, candidiasis), treatment is a long-term project. In a typical case a patient consulted a holistic practitioner after taking a long course of antibiotics during convalescence after surgery. The therapist responded by testing the blood for Candida. The lab report showed yeast-like particles in the blood. The therapist immediately started the patient on a course of garlic juice, and then aloe vera juice. Then he repopulated the intestine with Lactobacillus acidophilus tablets along with a milk-vegetarian, low carbohydrate diet. He used herbs, vitamins and a careful exercise and sunlight regime to restore the patient's immunity.

A consistent and special diet can often clear up all the residues of antibiotics as well as yeast infections and other side effects, provided it is well managed. Andrea, a 27-year-old actress and dancer suffered from a bladder infection three and a half years ago. She was given antibiotics for three to four weeks and then another course for a similar period. She developed yeast infections for which she was given powerful antifungal drugs. Since that time she has had regular bouts both of urinary infections and yeast infections, for which antibiotics were repeatedly prescribed. Meanwhile her physical and mental health worsened. Eventually she saw a gynaecologist for breast cysts who said that the antibiotics were not helping her. So she turned to a macrobiotic therapist. He gave her an 'Oriental diagnosis'. He told her that her immunity had been virtually destroyed by the antibiotics, and she was vulnerable to cancer. He put her on a strict macrobiotic diet. She went to cookery classes to learn how to prepare the food. The diet immediately cleared up the yeast and bladder infections. She concluded: 'I gained weight and lost it again, and started thinking clearer and feeling brighter. I have never had an antibiotic since.'

AIDS patients are particularly vulnerable to side effects because of the cocktail of drugs that need to be taken for long periods. The main drug is zidovudine ('AZT', 'Retrovir') which is an antiviral drug. The antibiotic trimethoprin-sulfamethoxazole (e.g. 'Bactrim', or 'Septrin') is also normally given prophylactically to prevent pneumonia and other infections. A range of other drugs are used. All these drugs produce a long and distressing list of side effects, largely on the skin, blood, spleen, liver and bone marrow. Naturopaths in the United States are building experience at treating these side effects. A variation of the nutritional supplement cocktail described above is used, emphasising vitamin E, folic acid, B6 and minerals. These help to protect the blood cells and restore deficiencies created by the drugs. In addition herbs are given to treat the kinds of symptoms described in the last chapter, such as Quercitin against rashes. Chinese herbs such as Dong Quai are utilized to protect the blood, liver, stomach and nerves from the drug-related toxicity.

Steroids

These drugs were introduced 40 years ago, and brought instant relief to arthritics. They include betamethasone (for instance, 'Betnesol' in the UK or 'Betacort' in the US), dexamethasone (for instance, 'Decadron'), prednisolone (for instance, 'Deltastab' in the UK, 'Cordrol' in the US) and others. I will let the American government's Food and Drug Administration tell you how they now see these 'miracle drugs' (FDA Consumer September 1985):

'Many patients quickly reverted to their previous condition when the cortisone treatment ceased. And – even worse – devastating and frightening side effects often accompanied cortisone treatment...side effects included insomnia, psychotic behaviour, growth suppression in children, peptic ulcer, delayed wound healing, hyperglycemia (excessive sugar in the blood), carbohydrate intolerance, muscle weakness, susceptibility to infections and many others. Surgeons reported deaths under general anaesthesia of patients under-going minor surgery who had been taking cortisone. In addition, cortisone proved to have a habit-forming potential – stopping the drug often brought on withdrawal symptoms...Where physician and patient alike had been attracted to the miracle of cortisone they were now repelled...'

Although I promised not to frighten off readers with side-effects stories, the situation with steroids is so scary that in this case I break the rules. Letters I receive tell a tale of anguish: 'How can I make love when my hips are crumbling?' 'Steroids cause fractures and weak bones, why use it for arthritis?' queries Babs Diplock, steroid victim and heroic campaigner. 'They cause muscle wasting and weakness. Why use for MS? They cause stomach pain, obesity and bowel problems. Why use for colitis? They cause cataracts and glaucoma. Why use for eye problems? They worsen asthma, so why use for asthma?'

The adrenal glands normally produce steroids to control stress, immunity, salt and water balance and other important functions. Taking steroid drugs short circuits these glands and after a while they give up. This makes any long term use of steroids hazardous. The only occasions which justify their use would be emergencies (allergic reactions, asthma crises, shock) or where the adrenal glands don't work, or in low doses to the skin, to tide you over a bad patch while you seek proper treatment. Steroids *are* absorbed through the skin.

Despite the problems, doctors still can't help prescribing steroids freely because it is so temptingly easy to stop symptoms in conditions like asthma, allergies, rheumatic and arthritic problems, eczema, and colitis. You should be aware that the disease will still be there (suppressed), side effects accumulate, and it postpones the search for a proper cure.

Alternative practitioners see many people who are on steroids. As long as there is some life left in the adrenal glands, a skilled alternative practitioner can unwind the tangle of steroid symptoms, eventually exposing the kernel of the allergy, eczema or asthma and treating that too.

Acupuncture is potentially valuable in restoring function to degenerated organs. It is able to channel energy to the organ like dredging a blocked irrigation channel so as to provide extra water for a parched crop. In acupuncture terms the damage to the adrenal glands is a deficiency of 'kidney yin', or internal energy. Treating the kidney yin points gradually restores the group of functions which it influences, including weak bones, thin skin, poor resistance to disease, waterlogging of the body and lack of energy and libido.

For example a 45-year-old woman came to see an acupuncturist after a pain clinic had given her a course of injections of steroids in her back against severe back pain. The specialists couldn't find any physical cause for this pain, which was unrelieved. But she had gained 13.5 kilos in weight, had a moon face, perspired constantly, was occasionally incontinent and trembled all the time. An adrenal test showed that the adrenal glands were hardly working. Her first acupuncture treatment was on May 5th at which several points were needled. She felt almost immediate pain relief but it came back after a few hours. She reported the next day, however, that it was the first time she had woken up without pain. Also her hands had stopped trembling. Within two days her perspiration stopped. On May 14th an adrenal test showed that the glands were 80 per cent normal, which is an unusually fast recovery. Treatment continued. She had longer and longer pain-free intervals. By the end of June she had lost most of her extra weight, and by mid July her pain had gone.

One of the acupuncturists I spoke to had weaned several patients off steroids. One patient was on high doses of steroids for systemic lupus erythematosus (SLE). He stepped down the dosage quite quickly with the help of acupuncture and diuretic/liver stimulating herbs such as dandelion. She improved and came off steroids completely in two months. Later she fell over backwards while dancing and shattered both her wrists – the bones were very brittle as a result of the steroids. The acupuncturist strengthened her repair processes which helped the fractures to mend. He stressed that the bones and the kidney can take up to a year to recover.

Children are very often given steroids for problems like asthma, eczema and allergies. Yet among the causes may be a disturbed, loveless home, stress, poor diet, poor immunity, not enough breast feeding. Homoeopathy does well with children, provided a good rapport is established, and the practitioner works with the family to examine the background to the problem. One homoeopath described a nine-year-old girl who came from a disturbed family. She had had asthma and eczema since she was a baby and had been on steroids since then. He treated her using various homoeo-pathic preparations – which in her case included pulsatilla, arsenicum, turbercullonium, zinc, and Bach flowers. She was able to stop taking steroids internally overnight and slowly worked her way off steroid creams over six months.

Other alternative practitioners would concentrate on diet and herbs. Vitamin B complex, C and E can, to some extent, protect the adrenal glands and the kidney, and extra potassium helps with the salt/water balance. Hormone-stimulating herbs can be used to replace the steroids gradually. Extra body water can be drained by herbal diuretics, while herbs such as meadowsweet can prevent the inflammations from flaring up again. There may be special promise in Chinese herbs such as bupleurum, hoelen and persica. A study at the Institute of Oriental Medicine in Osaka, Japan, looked at 52 patients who had been given long-term steroids for rheumatic, liver and kidney problems. It showed that side effects could be notice-ably reduced within three months and they could stop taking steroids after six months, providing they took these Chinese herbs regularly.

Non-steroid anti-inflamatory drugs (NSAIDs)

The side effects of steroids precipitated a rush to find other kinds of drugs useful against rheumatic and arthritic diseases. There is now a great number of such drugs, called Non-Steroid Anti-Inflammatory Drugs (NSAIDs). They do not act on the adrenal glands like steroids, but on local body messengers termed prostaglandins. They are the most widely prescribed of all drug categories. One in seven Americans are being prescribed these drugs now. They include the salicylate-aspirin type, which we will not deal with here, and non-salicylates such as ibuprofen (e.g. 'Nurofen' in the UK or 'Advil' in the US), indomethacin (for instance, 'Indocid' in the UK, or 'Indocin' in the US), naproxen (for instance, 'Naprosyn'), fenoprofen (for instance, 'Fenopron' in the UK or 'Nalfon' in the US).

These drugs were always thought safe, until, as time has gone by, worrying side effects have emerged. They affect the kidney, causing kidney failure, waterlogging of the tissues and poor general health. With long-term use the kidneys may suffer irreversible damage. A recent study by researchers at John Hopkins University found that one out of four women who already had mild kidney disease who took ibuprofen suffered kidney failure. They produce tinnitus, breathing difficulties, depression, chest pain. They cause stomach bleeding, indigestion and stomach ulcers by stripping the stomach lining, which can cause allergies or even life-threatening holes. 'From our evidence, all patients taking NSAIDs must be assumed to be at risk of developing peptic ulceration ... NSAIDs should be avoided whenever possible' stated a study in the *British Medical Journal* on 10th February 1990.

The tragedy is that these drugs merely treat symptoms. The underlying arthritic and rheumatic disease is not understood or treated by modern medicine. There are in alternative medicine many well-tried natural remedies for these problems. Dietary treatment is very effective. According to clinical studies at the Epsom District Hospital, UK, three quarters of rheumatoid arthritis patients got better just by changing their diet. Rheumatic diseases are helped by controlled fast and alkaline diets, low in refined carbohydrates and high in vegetables. Eat only cold-pressed not refined oils. Exclude solanaceous vegetables – tomatoes, aubergines (egg-plants) and potatoes. Exclude caffeinated drinks, alcohol, and sugar-containing foods and drinks. Take alfalfa and kelp supplements, vitamin C and B vitamins.

Herbal treatments include black cohosh, blue cohosh, Devil's claw, celery seed, parsley seed, green-lipped mussel, nettle and dandelion. The treatment is complex as at the root of arthritis may be allergic, liver or kidney problems which must be cleared up first. There are, however, many herbal anti-inflammatory remedies and external embrocations, which can relieve symptoms more safely than the NSAIDs.

The evidence is that aspirin is as good as most other NSAIDs and a very great deal safer. If you can, stick to aspirin. However if you are already taking other NSAIDs, there are a number of holistic treatments that can protect you. Aloe vera juice brings relief from inflammation of the stomach. Some initial research suggests that when taken internally it stops allergic reactions created by drugs, yeasts or holes in the stomach lining. You should consider taking aloe vera juice to protect the stomach from the effects of NSAIDs. It can also help with rheumatic diseases as a whole by reducing the inflammation throughout the body. The stripping of the stomach lining can be prevented or reduced by slippery elm, Irish moss, or other soothing 'demulcent' or mucilaginous herbs. After the drugs are stopped, liquorice in the morning before food will repair ulceration.

Gamma linolenic acid (GLA) may be a considerable help while dosage of the drugs is being reduced. It is itself of potential benefit to rheumatic or arthritic diseases, for GLA is one of the natural components of the prostaglandin chain that seems to be disturbed or deficient in these diseases. Although it cannot express these benefits during drug dosage since the drugs work in the opposite direction, research shows it can prevent drug side effects. Take GLA while reducing drug dosage, and continue afterwards. It can be obtained as evening primrose oil or blackcurrant seed oil capsules in health shops or chemists.

Vitamin E and vitamin C are known to reduce kidney damage caused by drugs, and can prevent scarring when the damage is repaired. The suggested dose is: vitamin E 400 IU per day, vitamin C one gm per day.

Blood pressure lowering drugs

An abundance of advertisements for blood pressure reducing drugs colour the pages of the magazines that doctors read. They may show a family man happily pottering about the house, with the broad hint that life can be wonderfully normal through these drugs. Doctors have been persuaded to prescribe them to perhaps two million people in the UK, at a cost to the National Health Service of about £120 million per year. Perhaps 15 million people in the US take them.

There are a great variety of these drugs, all working on different mechanisms. The beta-blockers such as propranolol (for instance, 'Inderal') block arousal messages from the nerves to the heart. Other drugs like hydralazine (for instance, 'Apresoline' in the UK or 'Apresazide' in the US) expand the blood vessels, others block pumping messages in the heart itself. Others stop the brain from overstimulating the heart, such as reserpine (for instance, 'Serpate', only used in the US) or methyl dopa (for instance, 'Aldomet'), and there are diuretic drugs which stimulate the kidney to get rid of extra water in the body. They are often used along with other drugs.

These drugs do have insidious side effects which, over time, can make you less and less healthy, active and lively. They frequently cause depression, tiredness and impotence. Artificially lowered blood pressure itself may lead to dizziness, nausea, cold and cramped hands and feet, tiredness, and digestive problems. The diuretics can harm the kidneys, and cause dizziness, headache, tinnitus, and eventually, bone problems. Once you start on these drugs, doctors will tell you, you are on them for life. Indeed it is hard to withdraw from them without risk to your heart.

To add insult to injury perhaps three quarters of all the patients who have been on these blood pressure lowering drugs do not actually need them. This came to light in the $100 million 'Mr Fit' study in the US, investigating which factors in the diet encourage heart disease. Nothing much of value emerged from the study except that those treated with drugs tended to have a higher death rate than any of the other groups making up this massive study. After much prodding the US National Heart, Lung and Blood Institute finally came out against drugs for raised blood pressure:

Patients with a diagnosis of mild to moderate hypertension should be encouraged to adopt non-pharmacological approaches as definitive intervention. That means, don't take drugs; rather, reduce weight, reduce dietary salt, get more exercise and unwind properly, which is, of course, what alternative practitioners have been saying for donkeys years.

A similar twelve-year study in the UK run by the Medical Research Council, covering 85,572 'patient-years', found that treatment did not save lives, and did not reduce the risk of heart attacks. Some 15 to 20 per cent of the patients had serious side effects. One stroke was prevented in every 850 people taking the drugs: a niggardly return for such widespread drugging. The medical establishment in the UK also concluded, in an Editorial in the *British Medical Journal* (Vol. 290, p. 322, 1985) that drugs should not be given in mildly raised blood pressure.

So, don't start on these drugs unless you have very high blood pressure. But do *something*, as untreated high blood pressure shortens life. First check that it is real, as blood pressure can be raised temporarily by any energetic or stressful activity. Get a proper diagnosis. Then treat it as a very useful warning rather than a problem, and get preventive help. Fortunately holistic management can sort out most mild blood pressure problems. This means progressive relaxation or meditation, a reasonable amount of exercise, and a fundamental change of diet, along with counselling to help manage the stressful forces in your life.

The main herbs are those for relaxing the nerves such as lemon balm or catnip, herbs for sweating such as elderflower or peppermint, those to increase the flow of urine including horsetail and juniper, herbs to reduce fats in the arteries especially garlic, and herbs to open the blood vessels and reduce blood pressure such as limeflower tea and hawthorn. If you decide that you really want to take blood pressure lowering drugs, the safest may be those based on the Indian herb Rauwolfia. This plant gave rise to the classical drug reserpine, but is now available from your doctor as a plant extract (for instance, 'Hypercal' in the UK or 'Raufola' in the US). At low doses it is safe; ask your doctor about it.

You can come off blood pressure lowering drugs with the co-operation of a doctor. He will provide a gradual step-down programme with constant checks on the way. But you must have alternative treatment at the same time.

Certain side effects of blood pressure drugs such as apathy, depression, lack of concentration, confusion, tremor, muscle weakness and twitches, tingling, cramps, loss of appetite, digestive disturbances and disturbances of heart rhythm may all be due to a lack of magnesium. Diuretics, especially, can drain the body of magnesium. Make sure your diet is rich in magnesium or take magnesium supplements. Magnesium salts such as magnesium sulphate (Epsom salts) are not well absorbed. However you can now purchase specially designed magnesium supplements containing magnesium aspartate, magnesium citrate or magnesium orotate. Take half a gram per day. Magnesium may even aid high blood pressure by itself. There is evidence that it works just like certain new drugs called calcium blockers. If you are prescribed these drugs, you may be able to achieve the same effect more safely by taking extra magnesium.

Impotence is reversible after stopping the drugs. It can be helped, according to Chinese researchers, by deer horn extracts (pantocrine) available in Chinese shops or supermarkets.

When taking diuretics you need extra B vitamins especially B6, magnesium, zinc and potassium. Of these only the potassium depletion will be recognized by the average doctor. He may give you potassium tablets. Be wary of them as they can cause stomach ulcers. Instead eat potassium-rich fruit especially apricots, bananas, cherries, grapes, raisins and citrus. The other minerals are obtained from a diet rich in nuts and seeds and green vegetables plus wheat germ, molasses and cider vinegar.

Keep taking a supplement called EPA, a polyunsaturated component of certain fish oils. It thins the blood, prevents blood clots and reduces the chances of a heart attack. There is such a sound backing of research for EPA that doctors are now prescribing it.

Over-the-counter (OTC) painkillers

Those people taking aspirin regularly might be forgiven, when they reach this part of the book, for hoping that I will leave good old aspirin alone! It is true that aspirin is much safer than the drugs we have been describing. However aspirin does have identical effects on the stomach to the NSAIDs just mentioned. Doctors looking into the stomach can always recognise aspirin users – the stomach lining may be raw and often bleeding. Aspirin may have other effects on the body including temporary infertility.

The medical attitude to aspirin has shifted. The UK Government's Committee on Safety of Medicines recommends that aspirin should not be given to young children with fever. The British National Formulary also states, *It is important to advise families that aspirin is not, in the evidence now available, a suitable medicine for children with minor diseases.* On the other hand they would recommend instead NSAIDs such as ibuprofen, which we have just identified as possibly worse.

In my view it is better to take aspirin than ibuprofen, provided you observe certain precautions described below to protect you from aspirin's attack on the stomach. It is better still to take herbal aspirin. In particular, willow bark extract contains the compound salicin, from which aspirin was originally obtained. It works like aspirin in the body but is safer.

Try not to take aspirin and similar drugs automatically to bring down fevers. Fevers rustle up your body's defences, increasing anti-bodies and white blood cells and helping to destroy viruses with the natural virus-killer interferon. If a fever rises, sponge with cold water and keep the head wrapped with cold wet towels. But seek medical help if it persists or gets very high.

If you have to use aspirin regularly:

- Take half a gram of vitamin C three times a day together with B vitamins, especially B6 and pantothenate. These vitamins help to restore the vitamin losses produced by aspirin. They protect the adrenal glands from being over-stimulated by aspirin and help to protect the kidney. Eat plenty of fruit, green vegetables and milk products to maintain sufficient calcium and potassium.
- Remember that aspirin thins the blood. Do not take it before surgery.
- Take aspirin with milk or food to reduce the effects on the stomach. Taking it with acid drinks such as fruit juices is more harmful to the stomach. Take slippery elm, linseed tea, or Irish moss daily to soothe and coat the stomach.

Paracetamol

The other common painkiller is paracetamol (e.g. 'Panadol' or 'Calpol' in the UK and 'Tylenol' in the US) and though this drug does not have destructive effects on the stomach it can affect the liver. An editorial in the *Lancet* (13/12/1985) stated that if paracetamol had been discovered today it would never have been allowed on sale without a prescription. For it is safe in low doses, but harmful in doses very little more than the recommended maximum dose of four grams per day. Only 6.3 grams per day has been found to be toxic to the liver, and paracetamol is one of the commonest causes of liver failure. When combined with aspirin it is potentially more toxic than either alone, and may also harm the kidneys.

Don't ever take paracetamol beyond the stated maximum dosage. If you are on a fast, if you drink alcohol regularly, if you have had hepatitis or have a weak liver, don't take any paracetamol at all.

Vitamin C, E, with sulphur containing amino acids (in egg yolks, garlic and onions) can help to break down paracetamol. However if an overdose is suspected seek hospital treatment with cysteamine immediately, even if there are no symptoms. The symptoms of liver damage appear after three to four days when it is too late to do anything about them.

If you have to take a painkiller occasionally, aspirin is still safer than paracetamol and ibuprofen.

Alternative practitioners should be consulted about any continuous pain if you have no better solution than continuous painkillers. Acupuncture is often very helpful. It can treat the pain and 'cool' a stomach 'heated' (that is, stripped) by painkillers. Alternative therapists with a trained eye may treat side effects of painkillers which you do not at first see, for example a dulled quality in the nervous system, which can make it harder to adapt to changes in the climate or personal circumstances.

Chapter Eight

BIRTH: PREVENTING RISK TO YOU AND YOUR BABY

A bright-eyed quiet, attentive newborn?

It was a windy Saturday afternoon in March 1977 when labour began. We were tremendously excited at the prospect of the birth of our first child. The contractions stopped as soon as we got to the hospital in North London, because, as my wife remarked, no one in their right mind would want to be born in such a clinical place. Then the farce began. The contractions restarted while we fenced off a series of authoritative suggestions: 'You ought to have an epidural anaesthetic now, it is much more difficult later on.' 'We want to see the baby's heart beat on the screen, don't you too?' which then turned into commands: 'Of course you must have a drip we cannot help you any other way.' I refused the staff. They refused me: 'No, you cannot turn off the fluorescents.'

Glaring lights, the monitor wheeled in and out, the nurses popping in at regular intervals 'to discuss the epidural'. Then: 'We must induce now, you have had long enough' and from a sister: 'Come on, it's Sunday morning.' While we were distracted by irritating medical debates the birth was induced. The contractions stormed. My wife screamed. 'Don't shout, you are disturbing others – you are not alone here you know!' The baby was taking its own time. The midwife came in: 'What? Still at it? If you haven't had the baby in five minutes we will use forceps.' 'Push!' 'I'm not ready!' 'Push!' Under threat, in pain, the baby was born.

We were all fine, but depressed at the loss of our birth.

Throughout this book we have been talking about risks and

benefits in relation to medical treatment that you are considering for an illness. Birth is different because it is not an illness, and any medical side effects are wreaked mostly on two healthy people, who are trying to carry out a natural, powerful and ultimately fulfilling act. This makes the side effects all the more serious. It is true that there is a very small percentage of high-risk birth cases, and birth is a risky moment in our life. This is the expressed reason for all the medical procedures and paraphernalia. But in order to justify itself, and in an excess of zeal, this birth apparatus tends to encompass every birth, normal or not.

Over the last 15 years a concerted campaign for natural birth has born fruit. You now have much more choice in the type of birth you want. Hospitals have moved over to consider the mother as a consumer and don't meddle quite so much in your birth. Many places invite you to prepare a 'birth plan' a scheme setting out how you want your birth to run. The difference was already noticeable by 1979 when we had our second child. What was regarded as my 'interference with staff' in 1977 was seen as 'parent's choice' in 1979. This time we requested beforehand to be left completely alone, which was respected. We went to hospital at first light and were home with the baby for breakfast.

Nevertheless the medical birth still predominates. Home births are extremely difficult to arrange in most western countries. In the US midwives are more or less forbidden to deliver at home, and in the UK many obstacles are put in the way of midwives who wish to work in the community. While in principle there is now more freedom, in practice the staff in your local hospital may still be unwilling, or unable to help a healthy person do a natural thing. Sometimes medical procedures are 'sold' by a hospital to parents as precautionary measures, which may seem quite reasonable. The majority of the population are still either ignorant of, or frightened of, natural birth and it may be medicine itself which has taken away their confidence. As one teacher of the Lamaze technique (which stresses psychological preparation for a fulfilling natural birth) told me: 'Your will is removed right from the prenatal checkups. Your baby is tested with equipment, you are introduced to pathology and the continuous feeling of risk: something may be wrong. The doctor makes out he knows more about you than you know about yourself. No-one will trust the mother right from the beginning, and soon she no longer trusts herself. From then on the mother becomes more or less a patient and it is only natural that she really is a patient at the birth.'

The baby, too, has an interest in the proceedings and medical staff are rarely sensitive enough to see what the baby gets out of a natural birth. As the editor of *Birth and Family Journal* writes: *The bright-eyed, quiet, attentive newborn, who is the product of a birth in which the mother was relaxed, constantly supported, fully mobile, unmedicated, delivered gently and quietly...is not recognized in hospital obstetrics. Most nurses and obstetricians actually believe we are talking nonsense when we talk about them.* The experts expect, instead, *A sleepy neonate, one who does not focus the eyes or follow objects and mimic faces, one who feels poorly, is hard to 'contain' or comfort and has few periods of 'quiet alert' state.*

It is my intention in this chapter to explain what medical procedures to expect and the risks and benefits of each of them. Then I hope to show you how to obtain the safest and most fulfilling birth.

The medical birth

The first thing to understand about a medical birth is that it sets out to protect, but because of its sledgehammer-to-crack-a-nut approach it often ends up by doing the opposite. The statistics tell you this clearly. Eighteen to twenty-two infants per 1000 die at birth in America, which offers the most medicalized births in the world. Yet only eleven to fourteen infants die per 1000 in Holland where half of the births are at home without a doctor present. In an American study of 2000 births at home or in hospital, there were 30 times more birth injuries in hospital, and six times more neurological damage.

A major new study published in the *New England Journal of Medicine* (28/12/89) surveyed 12,000 women who gave birth in birthing centres around the United States where non-medical natural birth is encouraged. Only 4.4 per cent had a Caesarean section (see below) compared to around 30 per cent in the US general hospitals. The conclusion is that birthing centres offer a 'safe and acceptable alternative to hospital confinement.' So what are the risks? Let us examine them one by one:

Ultrasound

This is one of the first medical items on the birth menu. It is now used almost universally during the antenatal period to check rate of growth, due date, normal structure and fetal heartbeat, which it does using high-frequency sound waves in a manner similar to radar. Doctors even encourage ultrasound so parents can have a snapshot of the baby and see its sex.

But there are still doubts about its safety. Laboratory studies have revealed that ultrasound can cause altered emotional behaviour, slower nerve development and low birth weight in animals. It is harder to test this with people. But research has shown more dyslexia (difficulties in recognizing words) among children who have been scanned in the womb. The International Childbirth Education Association believes ultrasound can affect behavioural and neurological development and the child's immunity. Doubts about the safety of ultrasound have made the Food and Drug Administration, the American Medical Association, and the Bureau of Radiological Health, in the US, warn doctors that it should only be used for sound medical reasons, for example to check up on vaginal bleeding.

Recently the American College of Obstetrics and Gynaecology, and other bodies such as the US National Institute of Child Health and Human Development, have summarised clinical research on whether there is any point in automatically giving mothers ultrasound. Their conclusion: it doesn't help the mother or the child. It is very clear from this that you should *only* have ultrasound for good medical reasons.

Abdominal Foetal Electrocardiograph (UK) or Electronic Foetal Monitoring (US)

These machines, which we will call EFM for short, are electronic versions of the stethoscope. They record the baby's heartbeat on a screen. They are usually attached to the scalp of the unborn baby with clips when the birth gets going. Hospitals want to do it to every baby and they say that the availability of this monitoring is a good reason to have your birth in hospital. However the machine is a substitute for personal care. It is the major cause of unnecessary Caesareans, since a blip on the screen makes the doctors nervous. An experienced midwife with the traditional ear trumpet would have known it was nothing. Caesareans are three to four times more frequent in births that are monitored. More than that, it is a source of interference and stress to the mother, making her feel that she is a patient and something is going to go wrong.

Again, recent research has overturned all the assumptions and now clearly shows that all this medical monitoring equipment is unnecessary. An official summing up of all the research to date (*New England Medical Journal*, 1/3/90) shows that EFM does not improve the chances even of high-risk babies, and does not improve the outcome of birth (measured by mental development) compared to the old-fashioned midwives ear trumpet. The only thing it did was increase Caesareans. In other words you can feel comfortable about refusing EFM monitoring, and relying on the skill of an experienced midwife with her ear trumpet.

The artificial induction and stimulation of birth

The mother is blessed with a complex natural timing mechanism to bring on labour when the baby is ready. The womb contractions that eject the baby are controlled by a hormone from the brain, oxytocin, as well as others in the uterus itself. If doctors don't want to wait for nature, they can give artificial oxytocin (for instance, 'Syntocinon') by a continuous drip into a vein. The doctor may also artificially 'break the waters' (rupture the membrane). This is not trivial. Indeed it is officially described (by the World Health Organisation) as a medical intervention which augments labour.

There are certain medical situations where induction is necessary. These include toxemia, diabetes, a very late birth (over two weeks past the expected date of delivery) or foetal distress. These would account for three per cent of all births. Instead ten to twenty per cent of births are induced or stimulated. The culprit may be ultrasound which gives the wrong date, based on machine time not natural time. When the date has passed the doctors get nervous and induce.

So what are the risks with induction? The obvious one is that if the baby is not ready and has to be kicked out by the obstetrician it may be premature, and this can harm the baby. Induction produces a 'tumultuous birth' – extremely strong and frequent contractions which are painful to the mother. They make you lose control of the birth and the baby can be damaged by the strong contractions. Also, the blood supply to the baby is reduced and the umbilical cord more likely to be compressed. If the dosage of hormone is a bit too high, a whole collection of tears, ruptures and haemorrhages could result.

These problems mean that induction is usually the open door to a trail of further medical procedures. For example painkilling medication is almost universal in induced births. Forceps are more likely and real or false alarms on the monitor lead to increased Caesareans. Moreover there is now good evidence that induction of labour may cause jaundice.

The birth position

There are certain things that you should not do lying immobile on your back, namely eating, drinking and having babies. Traditionally, midwives were well aware of this and a major item of their equipment was the birthing stool. There is evidence that squatting or sitting opens the pelvis, increases 'pushing', recruits gravity to help you deliver, and eases contractions. The sitting position is used in Holland where only four per cent of births require forceps, compared to the US where forceps are used many times more frequently. Sitting-and-moving births are up to one third shorter than flat-on-back births with less pain and complications.

Sitting births are now being used more frequently in the UK; however, there are still many hospitals where staff can't break old habits and automatically encourage the mother to lie. Also medical procedures such as drips and EFM all tend to immobilize the mother. In such cases lying flat on your back can be seen as a medical side effect.

Painkillers, anaesthetics and tranquilizers

During pregnancy the body's own painkillers (endorphins) accumulate in the brain and lead to a natural analgesia and a very pleasurable 'high' – the peak experience of childbirth. These endorphins may also help to initiate milk secretion and the first loving connection between mother and child. However anxiety, stress, fear, and loss of confidence all reduce endorphins and make childbirth more painful.

Knowing this, many more mothers could have a drug-free birth if they prepared themselves beforehand, made a decision not to have painkillers if possible, and were given the emotional support to pass through the experience using their own resources.

When you go to hospital someone will soon ask you what kind of painkillers you want. The choices are:

1 Narcotics, relatives of morphine, such as Pethidine ('Pethidine' is the name in the UK, in the US it can be 'Meperidine' or 'Demerol' brands)
2 A drug against nausea, a side effect of narcotics.
3 Anaesthetic such as bupivacaine (e.g. 'Marcaine') injected into the spine, in particular epidural or spinal block.
4 Gaseous painrelievers particularly 'Entonox' (nitrous oxide and oxygen).
5 Total anaesthetics in the case of a Caesarean.

Often the hospital anaesthetist will encourage mothers to have epidurals, since he himself believes in the great advantages of a pain-free birth. If the birth is likely to be more difficult, such as a posterior, breech or twins, the consultant can put strong pressure on mothers to have an epidural when three to four centimetres dilated 'just in case' of a Caesarean.

For the mother, drugs produce a dozy and out-of-touch state that makes it more difficult to manage the birth, which is more likely to be managed by others: 'It could make the difference between a nightmarish haze and an exalting – if not effortless! – experience.' As epidural anaesthesia stops most feeling below the waist, you are less mobile and cannot push the baby with the contractions. The birth therefore takes longer, and there is more chance of a forceps delivery and tearing.

All drugs cross the placenta and affect the baby. The baby is very sensitive to drugs. Birth is also the time when the baby's brain is developing at its fastest. The drugs act on the breathing centres of the brain and the baby may not have enough oxygen at the most critical moment of its life. Children born of drugged mothers tend to be more sluggish and unresponsive. In some cases they may have to have a drug (naloxone, brand name: 'Narcan') which cancels the effects of pethidine. They may not cry or breathe so soon. They show less attention, orientation and sharpness. The baby and mother seem to have less intimate contact and psychologists can notice these effects up to one year later. There is even research which has demonstrated slower growth after using narcotics like pethidine. Epidurals are less harmful than narcotics as the anaesthetic is not injected into the blood stream. Gaseous pain relievers are much safer than any of the drugs or anaesthetics.

The surgical birth

The episiotomy

Sedated, feet in stirrups attached to an intravenous fluid bag and a battery of monitors, the woman in labour is set up so well for surgery, an operation had to be invented so the scene wouldn't go to waste. Enter the episiotomy. There is a lot of truth in this jibe by Dr Robert Mendelsohn in his book: *MalePractice*. The episiotomy is the second most common surgical procedure in the Western world. Though it is said to ease the baby's head out of the birth canal, a study of 17,000 births showed that it offers no advantage. The *British Medical Journal* (vol. 289, pp. 587–90, 1980) reported that women with episiotomies had more pain and scarring than those with tears that happen naturally.

Caesarean section

Julius Caesar is supposed to have been born by surgery, so the modern technique of opening the mother's abdomen and removing the baby is called Caesarean section. It might have been so named because of the trouble the Caesars gave their mothers, for Caesarean section is no joke. You are usually given a total anaesthetic as for any major surgery, then shaved and painted with antiseptic. With an intravenous drip and a bladder catheter you are wheeled into the operating theatre. The abdomen and the uterus are opened, and the baby removed. It takes five to ten minutes, followed by 45 minutes of stitching. You start walking within 24 hours and if all goes well you should be out of the hospital after a week.

There are sometimes good reasons why a Caesarean is necessary to save the life of the mother or baby. These reasons include:

- 'Placenta previa': if the placenta covers the cervix or comes in front of the baby.
- Cord prolapse: if the cord comes down the birth canal before the baby.
- Severe toxemia: if the mother has high blood pressure and inability to clear waterlogged tissues.
- Virus infections of certain kinds.
- Separation of the placenta.
- Diabetes.
- Foetal distress, in cases where not enough oxygen is reaching the baby.
- Some cases of 'Cephalopelvic Disproportion (CPD)' where the baby is much too large for the pelvis.
- Some cases of abnormal position, usually the breech presentation, in which the baby is positioned buttocks first.

Now these reasons should at the most amount to four to five per cent of all births. In fact there was a time when if an obstetrician had more than this rate of Caesareans, his colleagues would tease him. Today the Caesarean rate is two to three times greater in Europe and four to six times greater in the US. This is partly the result of all the other medical steps in birth. As Dr Mendelsohn wryly remarks: *If immobilization of the mother, artificial rupture of the membranes, drugs, induction and foetal monitoring all fail to produce a convincing symptom as an excuse for a Caesarean, the doctor always has one card up his sleeve. He can shake his head sadly and blame the victim by telling the mother that her pelvis is too small.*

The great numbers of unnecessary Caesareans are also due to private medicine (it increases obstetric incomes), and to anxiety of obstetricians. Obstetricians, like most doctors, have little training and experience in *normality*. Further, obstetricians tend to assume that once a Caesarean, always a Caesarean. However the evidence is clear that a normal birth after a Caesarean is still safer than another Caesarean, and this is now the position of the National Institutes of Health.

The side effects of Caesareans are those of any major abdominal surgery (see Chapter 4). This includes risk of infection, blood transfusion and pain. In addition there can be lung problems ('respiratory distress syndrome') or prematurity in the newborn and side effects of anaesthetics which may inhibit breast feeding. The commonest side effect is depression. The majority of mothers report a feeling of helplessness, depression, failure and perhaps some guilt because they had no active part in the delivery.

The special care unit

If the baby has breathing or other problems or is particularly premature it may be whisked off to a Special Care Baby Unit (SCBU) in the UK or Neonatal Intensive Care Unit (NICU) in the US. In some hospitals one in four or one in five babies are put in these twilight zones, at risk from infections, enclosed in incubators, attached to machines, and separated from mothers' contact and breast. But many babies are there because of complications arising from induction, painkillers, forceps, and artificially breaking the bag of waters. A study in the UK has shown that after breaking the waters and artificial induction babies are four to six times more likely to be in special units than after natural spontaneous birth.

There is no doubt that in serious cases of prematurity or foetal distress the special care unit can save lives. Yet only 15 per cent of underweight babies are sent to the units after home births, compared with 70 per cent of those in obstetric wards of hospitals, and the results are the same. In fact UNICEF reports that the world-famous obstetrician Dr Caldeyro-Barcia packs premature babies under their mothers' clothes next to her skin, with ample breast milk, and saves 90 per cent of premature babies weighing from 1 to 1.5 kilos, a statistic better than that of the Special Care Units.

Special Care Units can involve many procedures and strong drugs such as dopamine whose long term consequences have never been properly evaluated. Suction tubes, UV lights against jaundice, intravenous fluids, diuretics and so on can all cause side effects to heart, lungs and brain of the tiny infant.

How best to cope with a hospital birth

Preparation

It will be of great help to you to assume that your birth will be a normal, natural and fulfilling experience. Even if it seems inconceivable that this little pelvis will accept the baby, that these breasts will actually produce milk, or that this mind could ever suffer the pain of childbirth, you can assume that your body will rise to the occasion. This confidence keeps anxieties at bay, both yours and the medical staff's, and is a major defence against unnecessary medical treatment.

Another useful attitude is that it is your *own* birth, your own baby. Just as doctors did not take over the intercourse which conceived the baby, there is no reason why they should take over your delivery of the baby which was conceived. It is essentially a personal, private experience, involving you and your partner or helper only. Why should you let it out of your hands?

Along with your attitude of confidence your body *must* be in good shape. There is no point in choosing natural childbirth, creating a whirlwind of objections in hospital, fantasizing about candles, cushions and loving baths, if, when it comes to the birth you can't cope, and it all gets lost in a maze of medical machinations. So get fit! Eat a good nutritious diet with plenty of vegetables, and protein-rich foods, to make sure the baby grows well. Take lots of exercise, especially swimming, yoga and walking.

Midwives will be far more accommodating and helpful to you in arranging a natural birth if they see you are not coming in too soon (you should wait until the cervix is already a bit dilated), you are strong and fit, and you are coping well. It also helps if you are friendly and not hostile to the midwives and staff. Everyone will feel confident that it is going well. The staff will help you with your natural childbirth plans and leave you to get on with it.

You should get informed. There are several good books (see bibliography) and go to childbirth classes and preparation groups. They should teach you exercises, breathing and relaxation. They should teach you how to do without painkillers. But you should also learn about the medical side so that you won't be distracted or disturbed too much by the hospital habits.

Where to go for your birth? In the UK you would be recommended to go to a small GP unit, staffed by GPs, rather than to the obstetric unit of a larger hospital under the care of a specialist. The GP units produce less complications and you will benefit from your existing connection with your own doctor – and so will he or she. Small local or cottage hospitals will be better than big-city teaching hospitals.

In the US the best places to go are alternative birth centres, where the birth will be supervised by midwives with a doctor standing by. Failing that, seek a hospital with a family birthing room. The hospitals have seen a commercial opportunity in accommodating to the consumer demand for birth as a more family-oriented and less medicalized experience. They have introduced birthing rooms in which a more or less natural birth is possible. However they have severely discriminated against midwives, and you may find the birth still managed by a male doctor with all the attendant offerings of medical procedures.

You may be tempted to go to private medical care, since you will be given greater freedom and more personal attention and comfort. But be warned. Private medicine sells medical care, which is just what you are trying to avoid. There tends to be more medical interference.

Of course hospitals and birth centres change, depending on the attitude and personality of the obstetricians and doctors. You may find an enlightened obstetrician even in the biggest hospital, with an excellent reputation for the encouragement of natural birth. This information is usually available from local childbirth groups. Choose a doctor with a reputation for assisting home births and normal births, and without a reputation for Caesareans. The doctor should preferably be a family practitioner, if not, an obstetrician, and lastly a gynaecologist.

In all medicine, especially birth, the doctor is providing you a service. He is only necessary to the extent that you need him. In birth he may be especially unnecessary. The Head of Obstetrics at one of Amsterdam's main hospitals commented that in his experience only three to five per cent of all births need a doctor in attendance. Otherwise it can be safely left to the midwife. When you talk to a doctor to check out his unit, here are some questions:

■ Can he arrange for a midwife to attend the birth?
■ If the birth is going well is he prepared to leave it all to the midwife?
■ Does he support and agree with self-sufficient and natural birth?
■ Does he encourage fathers' participation and is this encouraged by the hospital where he works?
■ Is he prepared not to use electronic monitoring devices unless there are problems?
■ Does he give the labour the time it needs?
■ Is he experienced at vaginal delivery for a breech baby?
■ What is his attitude to epidural (spinal) anaesthesia and narcotics?
■ Does the hospital leave the baby with the mother straight after birth and at all times?
■ (If a high risk birth.) Will I be allowed to go into labour naturally should a Caesarean prove necessary?

The high-risk pregnancy

Most of the difficult births are known about beforehand. So supposing you are in a high-risk category and can perhaps expect a difficult birth or Caesarean. What should you do? Here are some common problems and ideas on how to deal with them before the birth.

Breech birth

Only three to four per cent of pregnancies result in a breech presentation, in which the baby attempts to come out bottom or feet first. It is a common reason for a Caesarean, but there are no hard and fast rules and successful vaginal birth is possible depending on the size and shape of the pelvis and cervix, the weight of the baby, how the labour is going, and the kind of breech position. The key lies with the doctor or obstetrician. Many are not experienced and will not hear of a vaginal delivery of breech birth. However you can and should find others who are able to deliver healthy babies in the breech position without extra risk, after a careful evaluation of each case. The birth must not be induced.

The breech can sometimes be turned by postural exercise beginning at seven months. This involves relaxing for ten minutes twice a day on a hard surface with knees bent, and pelvis raised about 30 centimetres by a pillow. Some midwives and obstetricians can also turn the baby from the outside, but they must know what they are doing.

Acupuncture can help breech babies to turn. In China this is very frequently used and there are reports of an 80 per cent success rate using a very simple procedure. It often involves 'moxa', that is burning little cones of a certain leaf of a plant over an acupuncture point. Here is such a case described by a woman in London who wanted a home birth:

'At 38 weeks my second baby was still in breech position and my obstetrician, who felt sure that the baby would not turn, made no attempt to turn it himself. Not willing to take unnecessary chances, and knowing that a breech baby meant hospital birth, I went with my midwife to see an acupuncturist. Using moxa on my little toes on alternate feet was, to my mind, a little bizarre, but as he applied the sixth cone and I felt the heat from it, I simultaneously felt a sort of gravitational pull towards the baby. To everyone's amazement the baby's head moved from the right side of my stomach over to the left. At the end of the treatment, the midwife put her hand on my

tummy and gently moved the baby a little further round. I
then felt a most peculiar sensation as the baby kicked himself
the rest of the way round so that his head was in the right
position. The same night the head engaged. I was delighted.'

Small pelvis

The diagnosis of 'CPD' is an excuse for many unnecessary
Caesareans. Therefore if you are given this diagnosis and a Caesarean
is suggested you should seek another opinion from a more
experienced doctor. In many cases further tests such as ultrasound
and a detailed examination just before birth will show that adjust-
ments are being made by both the baby's head and the pelvic
structure to allow a normal delivery.

Vaginal birth after a caesarean

It is hard enough to keep your trust in your body during a normal
birth in hospital. For a second birth after a Caesarean it is harder,
as it didn't seem to work the first time round. Actually doubts and
fears are more of a hindrance to a vaginal birth after a Caesarean
than any medical risk. Choose a doctor who will be happy to escort
you through a second vaginal birth. Remember that the first
Caesarean may not have been necessary or, as in a breech, may
have been exceptional.

There may be one in five cases where a Caesarean becomes
necessary again, usually because of rupture of the uterine scar, but
this is not dangerous. At least you know that you have tried.

The best chances of success are:

■ If the reasons for your previous Caesarean are absent.
■ If you have a normal pregnancy.
■ If you have had a previous vaginal birth as well as a Caesarean
  birth.
■ If the surgical scar was a transverse one.
■ If you have been in continuous touch with a supportive
  practitioner.
■ If labour is normal without induction.

During the birth

Your companion

Continuous care during birth from a partner or companion has been shown to cut the length of labour, often by half, and lead to fewer Caesareans. Research reports have clearly shown that there is less pain and medication, and the quality of the experience improved. Indeed a PhD thesis from Brandeis University on this issue found that 'peak experiences' during a childbirth were reported only by women whose partners were with them. Massage, talking, loving and sharing the experience allows the mother to relax. It is also very important that the partner keeps disturbances and unnecessary medical interference at bay, so that the mother does not need to be anxious or on guard. She can concentrate, conserve her energy, and let go.

Familiarity

Personal knicknacks, pictures, your own clothes, flowers or talismans are important within the alien hospital environment. They may help you relax and concentrate. Try putting up a picture in which you can 'lose' yourself on the wall opposite you. My wife stuck a postcard of the vaulted stone entrance archway of University College, Oxford, which looks like a passage or birth canal, in front of her during one birth. She concentrated so hard on being inside this that the hospital 'vanished'.

Sustenance

Labour is exhausting. You may need a little nourishment on the way. You should have small sips of water or herb tea sweetened with honey. Refuse to have a drip inserted into your vein unless there are clear *symptoms* of exhaustion, or in high risk births (for instance, breech), or if induction is an absolute necessity.

'Speeding things up'

If you are informed that your labour is 'not progressing', you should be sceptical, at least initially, and request that you be left alone to get on with it in your own time. If the doctor advises an induction ask for more time and ask for a second opinion. Meanwhile here are some tricks:

■ Walk (especially up and down stairs), squat, change position, move about. This is the best way of getting things going.
■ Take a little sustenance as described above.
■ Relax yourself completely using slow steady breathing. Concentration on the breath, as in yoga, is effective in aiding the opening of the cervix.
■ The brain hormones which control labour can be stimulated by suggestion. In India a grain jar is broken and the grain slowly poured out, or a flower bud is placed by the mother so that her cervix will open as it unfurls. Your partner can take you through images of opening, releasing and breaking.
■ Sexual stimulation can hasten labour, again through the hormones. In Jamaica women are given a man's sweaty shirt to smell. Labour can be initiated and hastened by gently handling the nipples or by bringing another baby to suck.
■ Acupuncture is probably the most reliable of the alternative methods for hastening labour. It stimulates the uterus, bringing renewed energy to the whole birth process. Here is an account by a mother whose contractions ceased after 24 hours of labour. The doctor wanted to induce the birth but the mother insisted on calling her acupuncturist:

'When my acupuncturist arrives I feel calmer. I feel needles making connection. About every five minutes he takes my pulses and slightly turns the needles which are left in. I feel extra surges of energy from those points every time he does another set of manipulations. I begin to feel the increased energy flow centering on my pelvis area, and after 10 or 15 minutes I experience my first contractions...'

From an acupuncturist's point of view, there are very precise points involved but it needs experience to select the appropriate points for each case. The kind of technique used is illustrated by Jan Resnick, a UK acupuncturist, in the case of Chris, whose contractions were weak and intermittent:

'We went on to leave needles in the colon four, stomach 36 and spleen six points for 30 to 40 minutes. Chris felt a lot of sensation drawing on her womb, and within ten minutes contractions began to increase in strength and frequency. Our spirits rose as progress was initiated but within two hours everything slowed right down. So we tried a second treatment which included the ear points called "uterus" and "endocrine" plus other points which the Chinese refer to in this context as "promoting labour", "benefiting the uterus", "moving the blood", and "dilating the cervix and facilitating delivery". Chris responded as before, with an impressive surge of energy, stronger contractions and a further opening of her cervix... before we knew it we were in transition.'

There are herbs which are used in traditional medicine where labour is difficult or stuck. These include birthwort, squaw vine, wild ginger, myrrh and pennyroyal. Although it may be impractical to have a herbalist on standby, the latter two are available as essential oils for smelling or massage.

Pain

Your birth classes will give you instruction on natural methods of pain control including breathing, relaxation, imagery and massage. Massage the back firmly during a posterior birth (the baby facing and pressing on the mother's back) and use efflorage – light strokes on the abdomen – for an anterior birth. You will find that at the moment when you cannot bear it one more minute, the birth is almost over – you have reached the top and are going down the other side.

Hypnosis is, as we showed in Chapter 5, an effective way of controlling pain and it certainly can be used before birth. However the commonest alternative method is acupuncture. Here is one woman's account of her acupuncture experience, published in the *Birth and Family Journal*.

'We reached hospital at 6.30 p.m. At 7.30 the doctor came, examined me and announced I was 4.5 centimetres dilated and was not going home without a baby. My husband, Greg, cheered. At 10.30 p.m. the acupuncturist placed the first needle in my left hand, between the thumb and forefinger well up in the crevice that separates them. The needles are so thin that they would more properly be called wires...it is barely possible to feel them enter let alone any pain.

Next a needle was placed in each of my calves, then two were placed in each of my feet. They were placed slowly and carefully taking time out during my contractions. During this process I continued to practice Lamaze breathing. The entire procedure took approximately 20 minutes. The relief occurred at the end of this period...As soon as the acupuncture took effect, the resident anaesthesiologist asked me to compare contractions. I felt that the next four were reduced in pain by half.'

If you do take painkilling drugs during birth there is not much you can do to prevent the baby receiving them. At least you can be prepared for the baby to be a little slow in feeding and reacting. You can help yourself to overcome dopiness by washing the drugs out with plenty of drink, by taking B vitamins together with small nutritious high-protein and low-starch meals, and by taking stimulating herb teas such as ginseng (see Chapter 7).

A quick getaway

The hospital is not a particularly conducive place to begin your new relationship, nor to start the rhythms of caring. You can ask for a 24-hour discharge beforehand, providing you do not have six children and the washing up waiting for you. Some hospitals accept the so-called 'domino system' of antenatal and birth care; you deliver, have a cup of tea and leave, but you must have elected to be part of this system beforehand.

Caesarean section

You may have done your best, and prepared yourself well, but sometimes things go wrong, and if you are satisfied that a Caesarean is necessary on clear medical grounds, what should you do to reduce the risks? If you have time to prepare for it, follow the recommendations and suggestions given in Chapter 4 on surgery and anaesthesia. You can also get help from special Caesarean preparation classes and from the books described.

It is important for the health of the baby that you only go to the operating theatre *after* natural labour has begun. This reduces the dangers to the foetus of prematurity. Respiratory distress is *several times* less frequent when a Caesarean section is performed after labour has begun.

Ask for a low transverse cut in the abdomen, which is usually hidden after a while by pubic hair, and a transverse cut in the uterus. This cut has much less chance of breaking in a future normal birth than the vertical cut.

For the sake of the baby, don't take premedication, which is anyway less necessary than usual. Choose a spinal or epidural anaesthetic rather than a general anaesthetic. It has less side effects on both the mother and child, it permits the mother to have contact with and feed the baby straight after the birth, to share the birth with the father and to be more involved. There is evidence that it minimizes any depression and sense of failure. Indeed anything that keeps the mother more in contact with delivery, especially keeping awake for it, will help to prevent later problems of relating to the baby and feeling a failure.

The father can share the procedure, give support, alleviate any sense of helplessness and anxiety and hold the baby soon after birth. It is absurd to think that a strange nurse, with one or two kind words, can replace him. The father can help even if the mother is unconscious during a general anaesthetic: he acts as her eyes and ears during the event. It used to be a fear of obstetricians that fathers at any birth, let alone at a Caesarean, would get in the way, or faint, or sue. This has now been amply disproved and indeed the National Institute of Health now recommends fathers' presence at Caesareans since they found that it helps the mother to recover more quickly.

The best place to start breast-feeding is in the recovery room, immediately after the operation. There is no reason why you should not start straight away, despite any drugs or residual anaesthetics. If the colostrum (the clear liquid that precedes milk) does not flow and the baby does not suck so readily, do not see it as another 'failure' – it is more likely to be due to the drugs and the answer is to try again occasionally.

You should choose a hospital for your Caesarean which allows you to go into labour first, encourages breast-feeding, and has a reputation for flexibility and understanding. You should also make sure of 24-hour visiting by the father, a great deal of information from the staff, and a room with other Caesarean mothers. Check that the hospital does not automatically send Caesarean babies to Special Care Units.

Protecting your baby from medical side effects

You can assume that whatever you experience the baby will receive too, in good measure. What can you do to protect the baby from the stresses of treatment?

One of the best ways is breast-feeding on demand. Even if the baby seems sleepy and sucks weakly you can express (squeeze out) a few drops of colostrum for the baby. If it is in a Special Care Unit your milk is vital. The nurses will help and encourage you to give milk which can be expressed with breast pumps for a child in a Special Care Unit incubator. A study published in the *Lancet* has proved that fresh breast milk is the best medicine for newborns after difficult births. Babies in special care receiving fresh milk had half as many infections as those receiving pasteurized human milk or human milk and formula. Substitutes such as formula or sugar-water do more harm than good by making breast-feeding more difficult. A drugged baby, arriving after a violent birth, needs extra contact, nourishment, and warmth which breast-feeding on demand can provide. Breast-feeding rhythms can be established later.

Cracked nipples can be very unpleasant and put you off feeding especially if you are weak. This is due to sucking on the nipple itself rather than the entire areola with mouth agape. It is a matter of technique which the midwife or senior nurse should teach you. Cracked nipples should be treated with wheat germ oil.

Any drugs that are necessary will enter your bloodstream within minutes and leave within hours. So take it straight after a feed in consultation with the doctor. Just as drugs pass to the baby, so do vitamins. You can help your newborn after a medicated birth by giving it vitamins in your milk. You should take B vitamins, and vitamin E and C in the dosages described in Chapter 3. This is in addition to the vitamins the hospital will give the newborn. Doctors reported in the *British Medical Journal* that vitamin E supplements (unheard of by most paediatricians) given to premature babies improve their chances of survival. You should also drink a lot of fluid and eat nutritious food. In Ireland they give Guinness to mothers after birth to get the milk flowing!

Try to keep the baby out of Special Care Units if at all possible. Paediatricians (attending all premature births) will not normally send a healthy baby to an SCU just because it is a bit premature. However, there may be borderline cases where the baby is premature and a bit slow or sleepy; this is where your choice makes a difference. Keeping the baby next to your skin with free access to milk has been proved to be more effective than SCUs for low birth weight babies.

Bear in mind that when a baby is put in an SCU it may suffer psychologically from disconnection with the mother. So if your newborn is in special care for a real medical necessity, be its nurse. Do everything for it yourself. Express milk for it, feed it, even switch on the machines for it.

When you get home, and the baby is safely nested consider what you can do to remove any scars of a medicalized birth from both of you. Difficult or traumatic births, especially by forceps, can leave tensions in the baby which make it fretful. Small babies respond well to homoeopathic treatment for symptoms which may have arisen from medical interference of any kind, including drug side effects. Go to a homoeopath soon after birth. Osteopathy can help release these tensions, calm the baby and soften the 'body memory' of the birth. Osteopaths have found that mechanical distortions of the top of the chest and neck area can be caused by forceps and difficult births. It can disturb the nerves which control breathing, leading to childhood asthma. They are sometimes able to correct the mechanical distortions and cure the asthma.

Massage is also useful for this purpose. You can do it yourself. Use thumb and forefinger to massage the limbs and back gently. There are instructions in the books by the French natural childbirth pioneer F. Leboyer. Use a little inert oil such as almond or olive oil, but not aromatherapy essential oils unless under a therapists advice. Touch, contact and your love can do a great deal to restore a peaceful connection with your baby, letting the healing happen by itself.

Appendix 1

FURTHER READING

A Consumer's Guide to Avoiding Unnecessary Radiation Exposure.
Laws, P., Health Research Group, Washington, DC, 1974
A Gentle Way with Cancer. Kidman, B., Century, London, 1983
A Time to Heal. Bishop, B., Severn House, 1985
Acupuncture for Everyone. Lever, R., Penguin, 1987
Alternative Maternity. Wesson, N., Optima, 1989
Aromatherapy for Everyone. Tisserand, R., Penguin, 1988
A-Z of Alternative Medicine(UK), Abercorn Hill Associates, 105–9
    Sumatra Road, London NW6 1PL
Birth Reborn. Odent, M., Souvenir, London, 1984
BMA Guide to Medicines and Drugs. Henry, J. (ed.), Kindersley, 1989
Cancer and Leukaemia: An Alternative Approach. Vries, J.,
    Mainstream, 1988
Cancer: How to Prevent It and How to Help Your Doctor Fight It.
    Berkeley, G.E., Prentice Hall, NJ
Cancer: Your Life, Your Choice. Clyne, R., Thorsons, 1989
Childbirth with Insight. Noble, E., Houghton Mifflin, Boston, 1984
Confessions of a Medical Heretic. Mendelsohn, R., Contemporary
    Books, Chicago, 1979
Cured to Death. Melville K.A. and Johnson, C.R., Secker &
    Warburg, London, 1982
Detox. Saifer, P. and Zellerbach, M., Tarcher, J.P., Los Angeles,
    1984
Drug Free Pain Relief. Lewin, G. and Horn, S., Thorsons, 1987
Encyclopaedia of Natural Medicine. Murray, M., Pizzorne, J.,
    Optima, 1990
Garlic, Nature's Original Remedy. Fulder, S. and Blackwood,
    J.,Healing Arts Press, Rochester, Vermont, 1992

Gentle Giants. Brohn, P., Century, 1986

Gesundheit! Adams, P. and Mylander, M., Healing Arts Press, Rochester, Vermont, 1993

Ginseng. Fulder, S., Thorsons, UK, 1989

Healing. Macmanaway, B., Thorsons, UK, 1983

Health Defence. Shreeve, C., David & Charles, 1987

Health Shock. Weitz, M., David & Charles, London, 1980

Herbal Medicine. Weiss, R.F., Beaconsfield Publishers, Beaconsfield, UK, 1988

Holistic First Aid. Nightingale, M., Optima, 1988

Homoeopathy for Everyone. Gibson, S. and R., Penguin, 1987

How to Choose a Good Doctor. Lemaitre, G.D., Andover, US, 1979

How to Fortify Your Immune System. Dickenson, D., Arlington Books, London, 1982

How to Meditate. Lawrence Leshan, Crucible, 1989

Hypnosis and Hypnotherapy, a Patient's Guide. Karle, H.W.A., Thorsons, 1988

I'm Dancing as Fast as I Can. Gordon, B., Harper and Row, NY, 1979

Limits to Medicine. Illich, I., Penguin, London, 1977

Loving Medicine. Patients Experiences of Personal Transformation through the Holistic Treatment of Cancer. Thompson, R., Gateway, 1989

MalePractice. Mendelsohn, R., Contemporary Books Inc., Chicago, 1981

Mind Over Medicine. Blake, R., Pan, 1987

Naturebirth. Brooks, D., Heinemann, London, 1985

Nutritional Influences on Illness. Wehrbach, M.R., Thorsons, 1989

Out of the Earth. Mills, S., Viking Penguin, New York, 1991

Patients Rights. National Consumer Council, HMSO, London, 1983

Peace of Mind. Gawler, Dr Ian, Prism, 1989

Planning for a Healthy Baby. Barnes, B. and Bradley, S.G., Ebury, London, 1989

Relief without Drugs. Meares, A., Fontana, London, 1983

Stress and Relaxation. Madders, J., Macdonald Optima, 1989

Take this Book to Hospital with You. Inlander, C.B., Weiner, E., People's Medical Society, Rodale Press, PA, 1985

The British National Formulary. British Medical Association, The Pharmaceutical Press, 1990

The Cancer Prevention Diet. Kushi, Michio and Jack, A., Thorsons, Harper Collins, London, 1988

The Complete Book of Massage. Maxwell-Hudson, C., Dorling Kindersley, 1988

The Complete Relaxation Book: A Manual of Eastern and Western Techniques. Hewitt, J., Rider, 1988

The Diseases of Civilisation. Inglis, B., Hodder and Stoughton, London, 1981

The Dr Moerman Cancer Diet. Jochems, R., Sheldon Press, 1989

The Handbook of Complementary Medicine. Fulder, S., Coronet, London, 1987

The Herb Society's Complete Medicinal Herbal. Ody, P., Dorling Kindersley, London, 1993

The Medical Risks of Life. Lock, S. and Smith, T., Penguin, 1976

The Natural Family Doctor. Stanway, A., Century Hutchinson, 1987

The New Good Birth Guide. Kitzinger, S., Penguin, London, 1983

The Practical Encyclopaedia of Natural Healing. Bricklin, M., Rodale Press, Emmaus, Pennsylvania 1990

The Relaxation Response. Benson, H., Morrow, NY, 1976

The Role of Medicine. McKeown, T., Nuffield Provincial Hospital Trust, London, 1976

The Whole Health Manual. Holford, P., Thorsons, 1988

The Wound and the Doctor. Bennet, G., Secker & Warburg, 1987

Thorsons Guide to Medical Tests. Trevelyan, J., Dowson, D., West, R., Thorsons, 1989

Total Massage. Hofer, J., Grosset and Dunlop, NY., 1976

Towards a New Science of Health. Lafaille, R. and Fulder, S., Routledge, London and New York, 1993

Traditional Medicine. World Health Organisation, Geneva, 1988

Vaccination and Immunisation, Dangers, Delusions and Alternatives. Chaitow, L., C.W. Daniel, 1987

Vitamin Robbers. Mindell, E. and Lee, W.H., Keats, New Canaan, 1983

When to Say No to Surgery. Schneider, R.G., Prentice Hall, Englewood Cliffs, NJ, 1982

Who's Having Your Baby? Beech, B.L., Camden Press, 1987
Worst Pills, Best Pills. Health Research Group. 2000 P Street NW,
   Suite 700, Washington, DC, 20036, USA
Your Health, Your Choice. Mills, S. (ed.), Macmillan, 1989

Appendix 2

USEFUL ADDRESSES IN THE UK

ACTION FOR VICTIMS OF MEDICAL ACCIDENTS
Bank Chambers, 1 London Road,
Forest Hill, London SE23 3TP
0181–291 2793

ACTIVE BIRTH CENTRE (INTERNATIONAL CENTRE FOR ACTIVE
    BIRTH)
55 Dartmouth Park Road,
London NW5 1SL
0171-267 3006

ARTHRITIC ASSOCIATION
122 Three Bridges Road,
Crawley, W. Sussex
01293-22041

ASSOCIATION FOR IMPROVEMENT IN THE MATERNITY SERVICE
    (AIMS)
163 Liverpool Road,
London N1 0RF
0171-278 5628

ASSOCIATION OF COMMUNITY HEALTH COUNCILS FOR
    ENGLAND AND WALES
30 Drayton Park,
London N5 1PB
0171-609 8405

ASSOCIATION OF PARENTS OF VACCINE DAMAGED CHILDREN
2 Church Street,
Shipston-on-Stour,
Warwickshire, CV36 4AP
01608-61595

ASSOCIATION OF RADICAL MIDWIVES
62 Greetby Hill,
Ormskirk, Lancashire L39 2DT
01695-72776

BACUP (BRITISH ASSOCIATION OF CANCER UNITED PATIENTS)
121–123 Charterhouse Street,
London EC1M 6AA
0171-608 1661
Freeline 0800-181199 for callers outside London.

BREAST CARE AND MASTECTOMY ASSOCIATION OF GREAT
   BRITAIN
26a Harrison Street,
London WC1H 8JG
0171-837 0908

BRITISH ACUPUNCTURE ASSOCIATION AND REGISTER
22 Hockley Road,
Raleigh, Essex SS6 8EB
0171-834 1012
0171-834 3353

BRITISH ASSOCIATION FOR COUNSELLING
37a Sheep Street, Rugby,
Warwickshire CV21 3BX
01788-78328/9

BRITISH ASSOCIATION OF HOLISTIC HEALTH
179 Gloucester Place,
London NW1 6DX
0171-262 5299

BRITISH CHIROPRACTIC ASSOCIATION
Premier House, 10 Greycoat Place,
London SW1P 1SB
0171-222 8866

BRITISH DIABETIC ASSOCIATION
10 Queen Anne Street,
London W1M 0BD
0171-323 1531

BRITISH HERBAL MEDICINE ASSOCIATION
Field House, Lye Hole Lane, Redhill,
Bristol, Avon BS18 7TB
01934-862994

BRITISH HOMOEOPATHIC ASSOCIATION
27a Devonshire Street,
London W1N 1RJ
0171-935 2163

BRITISH HYPNOTHERAPY ASSOCIATION
1 Wythburn Place,
London W1H 5WL
0171-723 444 (24 hours)

BRITISH MEDICAL ACUPUNCTURE SOCIETY
Newton House, Newton Lane,
Witley, Warrington WA4 4JA
01925-73727

BRITISH SOCIETY FOR NUTRITIONAL MEDICINE
PO Box 3AP,
London W1A 3AP
0171-436 8532

BRITISH TINNITUS ASSOCIATION
c/o Royal National Institute for the Deaf,
105 Gower Street, London WC1E 6AH
0171-387 8033 ext 201
0171-436 7637 (direct line)

BRITISH WHEEL OF YOGA
1 Hamilton Place, Boston Road,
Sleaford, Lincs NG34 7ES
01529-306851

CAESAREAN SUPPORT GROUP
81 Elizabeth Way,
Cambridge CB4 1BQ
01223-314211

CANCER HELP CENTRE
Grove House, Cornwallis Grove,
Clifton, Bristol BS8 4PG
01272-743216

CANCERLINK
17 Britannia Street,
London WC1X 9IN
0171-833 2451

CHEST, HEART AND STROKE ASSOCIATION
Tavistock House, North Tavistock Square,
London WC1H 9JE
0171-387 3012

COLLEGE OF HEALTH
18 Victoria Park Square,
London E2 9PF
0181-980 6263

COUNCIL FOR COMPLEMENTARY AND ALTERNATIVE MEDICINE
179, Gloucester Place,
London NW1 6DX
0171-724 9103

CYSTITIS AND CANDIDA
75 Mortimer Road,
London N1 5AR
0171-249 8664
Contact Angela Kilmartin

FAMILY HEART ASSOCIATION
PO Box 116, Kidlington,
Oxford OX5 1DT
018675-79125

GUILLAIN BARRE SYNDROME SUPPORT GROUP
Foxley, Holdingham,
Sleaford, Lincs NG34 8NR
Contact Glennys Sanders

HEALTH RIGHTS
344 South Lambeth Road,
London SW8 1UQ
0171-720 9811/2

HEALTH INFORMATION TRUST
18 Victoria Park Square,
London E2 9PF
0181-980 4848

HYSTERECTOMY SUPPORT GROUP
11 Henryson Road, Brockley,
London SE4 1HL
081-960 5987
0171-251 6332 (for name of local contact)

INTERNATIONAL STRESS AND TENSION CONTROL SOCIETY
The Priory Hospital,
Priory Lane,
London SW15 5JJ

INTRACTABLE PAIN SOCIETY OF GREAT BRITAIN AND
    NORTHERN IRELAND
9 Bedford Square,
London WC1B 3RA
Contact Dr. A.W. Diamond

LA LECHE LEAGUE OF GREAT BRITAIN
Box BM3424,
London WC1 6XX
0171-242 1278

MIND (NATIONAL ASSOCIATION FOR MENTAL HEALTH)
22 Harley Street,
London W1N 2ED
0171-637 0741

MYALGIC ENCEPHALOMYELITIS (ME) ASSOCIATION
PO Box 8, Stanford-le-Hope,
Essex SS17 8EX
01375-642466 (Mon–Fri 9am–5pm)

NATIONAL ASSOCIATION FOR PATIENT PARTICIPATION
Flat 6, Lansdowne, 1 Sydney Road,
Guildford, Surrey GU1 3LJ
01483-65882

NATIONAL ASSOCIATION FOR THE WELFARE OF CHILDREN IN
    HOSPITAL (NAWCH)
Argyle House, 29–31 Euston Road,
London NW1 2SD
0171-833 2041

NATIONAL ASSOCIATION OF HOMOEOPATHIC GROUPS
Alma Cottage, Brainsmead, Cuckfield,
West Sussex RN17 5EY
01444-458853

NATIONAL BACK PAIN ASSOCIATION
31–33 Park Road, Teddington,
Middx TW11 0AB
0181-977 5474/5

NATIONAL CHILDBIRTH TRUST (NCT)
Alexandra House, Oldham Terrace,
London W3 6NH
0181-992 8637

NATIONAL COUNCIL OF PSYCHOTHERAPY AND
   HYPNOTHERAPY REGISTER
c/o Stream Cottage, Wish Hill,
Willingdon, East Sussex BN20 9HQ
01323-501540

NATIONAL FEDERATION OF KIDNEY PATIENTS' ASSOCIATION
Acorn Lodge, Woodsetts,
nr Worksop S81 8AT
01909-562703

NATIONAL FEDERATION OF SELF-HELP ORGANISATIONS
150 Townmead Road,
London SW6 2RA
0171-731 8440

NATIONAL FEDERATION OF SPIRITUAL HEALERS
Old Manor Farm Studio, Church Street,
Sunbury-on-Thames, Middx TW16 6RG
01932-73164

NATIONAL INSTITUTE OF MEDICAL HERBALISTS
9, Palace Gate,
Exeter EX1 1JA
01392- 426022

NATIONAL REGISTER OF HYPNOTHERAPISTS AND
   PSYCHOTHERAPISTS
National College of Hypnosis and Psychotherapy,
12, Cross Street, Nelson, Lancs BB9 7EN
01282-699378

NEW APPROACHES TO CANCER
c/o Park Attwood Clinic,
Trimpley, Bedley, Worcs DY12 1RE
012997-375

NUTRITION ASSOCIATION,
36 Wycombe Road,
Marlow, Bucks SL7 3HX

PATIENTS ASSOCIATION
18 Victoria Park Square, Bethnal Green,
London E2 9PF
0181-981 5676
0181-981 5695

THE RELAXATION SOCIETY,
St. Mary Woolnoth Church,
Lombard Street,
London EC3V 9AN

RELAXATION FOR LIVING
29 Burwood Park Road,
Walton-on-Thames,
Surrey KT12 5LH

STEROID AID GROUP
PO Box 220,
London E17 3JR

TRADITIONAL ACUPUNCTURE SOCIETY
c/o Registrar and Secretary,
1 The Ridgeway,
Stratford-upon-Avon, Warwicks CV37 9JL
01789-298798

TRANX (UK) LTD
National Tranquilliser Advice Centre, 25a Masons Avenue,
Wealdstone, Harrow, Middx HA3 5AH
0181-427 2065
0181-427 2827 (24 hour answering machine)

WOMEN'S HEALTH CONCERN
PO Box 1629,
London W8 6AU
0171-602 6669

YOGA FOR HEALTH FOUNDATION
Ickwell Bury,
nr Biggleswade,
Beds SG18 9ES

Appendix 3

USEFUL ADDRESSES IN THE USA

AMERICAN INSTITUTE OF HOMEOPATHY,
1500 Massachusetts Ave., N.W.,
Washington, DC. 20005,

ACUPUNCTURE INSTITUTE,
9835 Sunset Drive, Suite 206,
Miami, FL. 33173,

AMERICAN INSTITUTE OF HYPNOTHERAPY,
1805 East Garry Ave., Suite 100,
Santa Ana, CA. 92705,

INTERNATIONAL HEALTH FOUNDATION,
PO Box 3494,
Jackson, TN

AMERICAN IMAGERY INSTITUTE,
PO Box 13453,
Milwaukee, WI. 53213

INTERNATIONAL FOUNDATION FOR HOMEOPATHY,
2366 Eastlake Ave. East,
Seattle, WA. 98102

NATIONAL WELLNESS INSTITUTE,
South Hall,
1319 Fremont St.,
Stevens Point, WI. 54481

AMERICAN HOLISTIC HEALTH ASSOCIATION,
PO Box 17400,
Anacheim, CA. 92817-7400

ASSOCIATION OF HOLISTIC PRACTITIONERS
6826 Chrysler St.,
Indianapolis, IN. 46268

AMERICAN ASSOCIATION OF ACUPUNCTURE,
Suite 601, 1424 18th St.,
Washington, DC. 20036

THE COMPLEMENTARY MEDICINE ASSOCIATION,
4649 E. Malvern,
Tucson, AZ. 85711

NATIONAL CENTER FOR HOMEOPATHY,
1500 Massachusetts Ave., NW 42,
Washington, DC. 20005

NETWORK CHIROPRACTIC,
1323 Anderson Ave.,
Fort Lee, NJ. 07024

HEALTH ASSOCIATION,
3301 Alta Arden, Suite 3,
Sacremento, CA. 95825

INTERNATIONAL FOUNDATION FOR HOMEOPATHY,
Suite 301,
2366 Eastlake Ave. E.,
Seattle, WA. 98102

HOMEOPATHIC ACADEMY OF NATUROPATHIC PHYSICIANS,
11231 SE Market St.,
Portland, OR. 97216

THE AMERICAN MASSAGE THERAPY ASSOCIATION,
PO Box 1270,
Kingport, IN. 37662

Mr. Charles B. Inlander,
PEOPLE'S MEDICAL SOCIETY,
462 Walnut St.,
Allentown, PA. 18102

AMERICAN ASSOCIATION OF NATUROPATHIC PHYSICIANS,
PO Box 20386,
Seattle, WA. 98102

AMERICAN ALLIANCE FOR COMPLEMENTARY MEDICINE,
PO Box 1843, Univ Station,
Charlottesville, VA. 22903

FOUNDATION FOR ADVANCEMENT IN CANCER THERAPY,
Box 1242, Old Chelsea Station,
New York, NY. 100113

HOMEOPATHIC EDUCATIONAL SERVICES,
2124 Kittredge St.,
Berkeley, CA. 94704

APPENDIX 4

THE EVIDENCE: SCIENTIFIC REFERENCES

The first edition of this book was published in 1987 by Century Hutchinson, under the title *How to Survive Medical Treatment*. My intention in this first edition was threefold. Firstly to guide patients towards protecting their health while under medical care. Secondly to demonstrate to medical and other professionals the hidden damage created by modern medicine as seen from a holistic perspective. Thirdly that there is scientific support for natural ways to avoid this damage. For this purpose the first edition has 492 references! Each significant statement in the book was referenced. Those readers who need to see this scientific backing, should refer to the first edition. This current edition is directed more towards those who enter medical treatment. So only the major references are given, as below.

The references are roughly in the order in which the material to which they refer appears in the text.

Chapter 1
Inlander, B.C., Levin, L.S. and Weiner, E. *Medicine on Trial*, Pantheon, NY (1990)
Fulder, S. and Monro, R. The Status of Complementary Medicine in the UK: Patients, Practitioners and Consultations *Lancet* 2, 542–5 (1985)
Eisenberg, D.M. et al., Unconventional Medicine in the United States *The New England J. of Medicine* 328 246–52 (1993)
Wharton, R. and Lewish, G. *Brit. Med. J.* 292, 1498–1500 (1986)
Hunt, S. M. et al. *J. Psychosom. Res.* 28 105–14 (1984)

Chapter 2

Cochrane, A.L. *Effectiveness and Efficiency*, Nuffield Provincial Hospital Trust (1972)

Graham, N.G. et al. *Brit. Med. J.* 2, 741–8 (1971)

Bennett, G. *Patients and their Doctors*, Balliere, Eastbourne (1983)

Pendleton, D. *The Consultation: An Approach to Learning and Understanding*, OUP, Oxford (1984)

Bradwell, A.R. *Lancet* 2, 1071 (1974)

World Health Organization Technical Report Series No. 689

Laws, P. *Medical and Dental X-rays: A Consumer's Guide to Avoiding Unnecessary Radiation Exposure*, Health Research Group, Washington, DC (1974)

The National Academy of Sciences, The National Research Council, *The Effects on Population of Exposure to Low Levels of Ionizing Radiation (Beir Report)* (1972)

FDA Drug Bulletin 30–31 (November 1978)

Tappel, *American J. Clinical Nutrition* 27, 960–5 (1974)

Cuckle, H. and Wald, N. Britain's Chance to Get Screening Right, *New Scientist* (15/10/88)

Wright, C.J. Breast Cancer Screening: A Different Look at the Evidence, *Surgery* (October 1986)

Chapter 3

Geiger, J. In Howard J. and Strauss, J. (eds) *Humanising Health Care*, John Wiley, NY (1975)

Feder, G. *Brit. Med. J.* 290, 322 (1985)

Falk, S.A. and Woods, N.F. *New Eng. J. Med.* 774–81 (11/10/73)

National Consumer Council, *Patients' Rights*, HMSO (1983)

David, T. et al. *Am. J. Phys. Med.* 39, 111–13 (1950)

Hartsfield, J. and Clopton, J.R. *Soc. Sci. and Medicine* 5, 529–33 (1985)

George, J.M. et al. *J. Behav. Med.* 3 (1980)

Fortin, F. and Kirouac, S. *Int. J. Nursing Studies* 13, 11–24 (1976)

Boore, J. *Prescription for Recovery*, Royal College of Nursing, London (1978)

Taylor, C.B. *J. Clin. Psychiat.* 43, 423–5 (1982)

Monro, R. *Yoga Biomedical Bulletin* 1, 29 (September 1985)

Bender, A. *British Medical J.* 288, 92–3 (1984)

Todd, E. et al. *Human Nutrition: Applied Nutrition* 38A, 294–7 (1986)

Robinson, G. et al. Impact of Nutritional Status on DRG Length of Stay, *Parent. Enter. Nutr.* 11, 49–51 (1987)

Steffee, W.P. Malnutrition in Hospital Inpatients, *Am. J. Clinical Nutrition* 33, 2595–600 (1980)

Editorial, *BMJ*, 212 (9 February 1974)

Irvin, T.T. *Surg. Gynaecol. Obst.* 147, 49 (1978)

Rasic, J.L. and Kurmann, J.A. *Bifidobacteria and their Role*, Birkhauser Verlag, Germany (1983)

Shorter, R.G. and Kirsner, J.B. (eds) *Gastrointestinal Immunity for the Clinician*, Grune & Stratton, NY (1985)

Shaw, D.M. *Br. J. Psychiatr.* 139, 580 (1981)

Dew, M. *Br. J. Clinical Practice* 38, 394–8 (1985)

Fulder, S. *The Book of Ginseng*, Healing Arts Press, Rochester, Vermont (1993)

Bieliauskar, L.A. *Stress and its Relationship to Health and Illness*, Westview Press, Boulder, Colorado (1982)

Chandra, R.K. *Nutrition Reviews* 39, 225–31 (1981)

Smith, R.G. et al. *Arch. Int. Med.*, 145, 2110–12 (1985)

Hall, H.R. *Am. J. Clinical Hypnosis* 25, 92–101 (1983)

Ding, V. et al. *Am. J. Acup.* 51–4 (1983)

Nordenstrom, J. et al. *Am. J. Clinical Nutr.* 32, 2416–22 (1979)

Chandra, R.K. *Am. J. Clin. Nutrition* 33, 13–16 (1980)

Horrobin, D.F. (ed.), *Clinical Uses of Essential Fatty Acids*, Eden Press, London (1982)

Bloksma, N. et al. *Planta Medica* 46, 221–7 (1982)

Center for Health Economics, *Economic Aspect of Hospital Acquired Infections*, University of York (1989)

Chapter 4

Editorial, *Lancet* 1, 593 (1979)

Weitz, M. *Health Shock*, David & Charles, Newton Abbot (1980)

Lewis, G.B. An Alternative Approach to Premedication: Comparing Diazepam with Auricular and a Relaxation Method, *Am. J. Acup.* 15, 205–14 (1987)

Goldman, L. *Awareness under Anaesthesia*, Ph.D. Thesis, Churchill College, Cambridge, UK (1986)

Hayward, D.J. *Information: A Prescription Against Pain*, Whitefriars Press, London (1975)

Clement-Jones, V. et al. *Lancet* 2, 946–8 (1980)

Herget, H.G. et al. *Der Anaesthetist* 25, 223 (1976)

Matsumoto, T. *Experimental Acupuncture Anaesthesia – Acupuncture for Physicians*, Charles C. Thomas, NY (1974)

Roscia, L. *Am. J. Chinese Med.* 1, 325 (1973)

Editorial, *Brit. Med. J.* 283, 746–8 (1981)

Solomon, et al. *Surgery* 87, 142 (1980)

Sung, Y.G. et al. *Anaesth. Analg. Curr. Res.* 56, 473–8 (1977)

Ceccherelli, F. et al. *Acup. Electrotherap. Res.* 6, 255–64 (1981)

Rodriguez, R. *Am. J. Acupuncture* 6, 123–6 (1978)

Stern, J.A. et al. *Ann. N. Y. Acad. Sci.* 296, 175–193 (1977)

Mckinlay, J. B. *Social Science and Medicine* 13A, 541–58 (1979). Subcommittee on Oversight and Investigations on Unnecessary Surgery (15/7/75)

Vianna, N. et al. *Lancet* 1, 431 (1971)

Lichter, and Pflanz, *Medical Care* 9, 322 (1971)

Editorial, *Lancet* 1020 (3/11/84)

Editorial, *New England J. Medicine* (2/7/82)

Editorial, *Lancet* 2, 1175 (1969)

European Coronary Surgery Study Group, *Lancet* 1, 889 (1976)

Editorial, *British Medical Journal* 1, 1163 (1979)

Bainton, D. et al. *New England J. Medicine* 294, 1147 (1976)

Editorial, *New England J. Medicine* 1249 (6/12/73)

Bunker, J., Barnes, B. and Mosteller, F. (eds) *Costs, Risks and Benefits of Surgery*, OUP, NY (1978)

Schmitt, F.E. and Woolridge, P.J. *Nursing Research* 22, 108–16 (1973)

Williams, J.L. et al. *Psychophysiology* 12, 50–4 (1973)

Boore, J.R.P. *Prescription for Recovery*, Royal College of Nursing, London (1978)

Shapiro, D.M., *Am. J. Psychiatry* 139, 267–74 (1982)

Hartsfield, J. and Clopton, J.R. *Soc. Sci. Med.* 5, 529–33 (1985)

Bradley, R.A. *Psychosomatics* 3, 1–6 (1962)

Hilgard, E.R. and Hilgard, J.R. *Hypnosis in the Relief of Pain*, Kaufmann, Los Altos, California (1975)

Wirth, D.P. et al., The Effect of Complementary Healing Therapy on Postoperative Pain after Surgical Removal of Impacted Third Molar Teeth, *Complementary Therapies in Medicine* 1, 133–8 (1993)

Johnson, J.E., and Leventhal, H.J. *Personal Soc. Psychol.* 29, 710–18 (1974)

Hill, C.F., Is Massage Beneficial to Critically Ill Patients in Intensive Care Units? A Critical Review. *Intensive Crit, Care Nursing,* 9, 116-21 (1993)

Barriga, J.D. Homoeopathy and Surgery, *J. Am. Institute of Homoeopathy* 143 (1975)

Bone, M.E. et al., Ginger in Postoperative Nausea and Vomiting, *Anaesthesia* 45, 669-71(1990).

Lobell, M.H. *Clinical Medicine* 69, 8 (1981)

Stevenson, C.J., The Psychophysiological Effects of Aromatherapy Massage Following Cardiac Surgery, *Complementary Therapies in Medicine* 2, 27–35 (1994)

Mullen, J.L. et al. Reduction of Operative Morbidity and Mortality by Combined Pre-Operative and Post-Operative Nutritional Support. *Annals of Surgery* 192, 604–13 (1980)

Irvin, T.T. et al. *Surg. Gynecol. Obstet.* 147, 49 (1978)

Editorial, *J. Am. Med. Assoc.* 137, 1228 (1948)

Van Druzen, R.E. et al. *J. Urology* 65, 1033 (1951)

Zucker, T.A. *Am. J. Clin. Nutrition* 6, 65 (1958)

Chapter 5

Palmer, V. et al. *British Medical J.* 281, 1594–7 (1980)

Brinklely, D. *British Medical J.* 288, 1709–10 (1984)

Cairns, J. *Cancer Science and Society,* San Francisco (1978)

Stoll, B. (ed.) *The Mind and Cancer Prognosis,* London (1979)

Meares, A. *Lancet* 978 (5/5/79)

Lerner, M. *Advances* 2, 31–43 (1985)

Cassileth, B.R. et al. *Annals Int. Med.* 101, 105–12 (1984)

Dundee, J.W., et al, Acupuncture Prophylaxis of Cancer Chemotherapy - Induced Sickness, *J. Royal Soc. Medicine.* 82, 268–71 (1989)

Dundee, J.W. et al., Non-invasive Stimulation of the P6 (Neiguan) Antiemetic Acupuncture Point in Cancer Chemotherapy. *J. Royal Society Medicine.* 84, 210–12 (1992)

Conway, A.V. *Holistic Medicine* 1, 43–5 (1986)

Newton, B. *Am. J. Clinical Hypnosis* 25, 104–13 (1983)

Mastenbrock, I and McGovern, L., The Effectiveness of Relaxation Techniques in Controlling Chemotherapy Induced Nausea – a Literature Review, *Australian Occupational Therapy J.* 38, 137–42 (1991)

Dempster, C.R. et al. *Int. J. Clinical Exp. Hypnosis* 24, 1–9 (1976)

Bridge, L.R. et al. Relaxation and Imagery in the Treatment of Breast Cancer, *British Medical J.* (5/11/88)

Ament, P.J. *Medicine* 13, 233–40 (1982)

Simonton, O.C. et al. *Getting Well Again*, Bantam, NY (1980)

Meares, A. *Austral. Fam. Physician* 9, 322 (1980)

Cameron, E. and Pauling, L. *Vitamin C and Cancer*, Warner, NY (1977)

Samachson, J. et al. *Arch. Biochem. Biophys.* 88, 355 (1960)

Razdan, R.K. and Howes, J.F. *Medicinal Research Reviews* 3, 119–146 (1983)

Yonezawa, M. et al. *J. Radiat. Res.* 26, 463 (1985)

Yuqing, X. et al. *Chinese Acup. and Mox.* 4, 6–8 (1984)

Salzer, G. *Onkologie* 1, 264–7 (1978)

Chapter 6

Boston Collaborative Drug Surveillance Program, *Paediat. Clins. North America* 19, 117 (1972)

Jick, H. *New Eng. J. Med.* 291, 824–8 (1974)

Melmon, K.L. *New Eng. J. Med.* 284, 136–41 (1971)

Hermann, F. and Herxheimer, A. In Soda, T. (ed.) *Drug Induced Sufferings*, Elsevier (1980)

Gershoff, and Priem, *Am. J. Clinical Nutrition* 20, 393 (1967)

Roe, D. *Drug Induced Nutritional Deficiencies*, Avi, Westport, Conn. (1976)

Ibid., *Nutrition Reviews* 42, 141–54 (1984)

Oversen, *Drugs* 18, 278–98 (1979)

Lancet 1, 929 (20/4/85)

Hsiao, et al. *Federation Proceedings* 34, 742 (1975)

Millard, P. *Brit. Med. J.* 289, 6452 (27/10/84)

Roe, D.A. *Drugs and Nutrition in the Geriatric Patient*, Churchill Livingstone, Edinburgh (1984)

Carrescia, O. et al. Silymarin in the Prevention of Hepatic Damage by Psychopharmacological Drugs, *Clinical Ter.* 95, 157 (1980)

Chapter 7
Committee on the Review of Medicines, *Brit. Med. J.* 280, 910–21 (1980)
Rawlins, M. and Smith, G. *Brit. Med. J.* 2, 447 (13/8/77)
Morgan, K. and Oswald, I. *Brit. Med. J.* 284, 942 (1982)
Teare, P.J. *Roy. Coll. Gen. Practitioners* 34, 258–60 (1984)
Vescovi, P. et al. Nicotinic Acid Effectiveness in Treatment of Benzodiazepine Withdrawal, *Curr. Ther. Res.* 41, 1017 (1987)
Editorial, *Brit. Med. J.* 705 (17/3/79)
Stein, E. and Stein, S.J. *Am. Geriat. Soc.* 33, 687–92 (1985)
Shader, R.I. and Dimascio, H. *Psychotropic Drug Side Effects*, Williams & Wilkins, Baltimore (1970)
Egan M.F. et al., Treatment of Tardive Dyskinesia with Vitamin E. *American J. Psychiatry* 149 773–77 (1992)
Moir, D. et al. In *Studies in Drug Utilisation*, WHO Regional Office for Europe, Copenhagen (1979)
Day, T.K. *Lancet* 2, 1174 (1975)
Berg, R. *Human Intestinal Flora in Health and Disease*, Academic Press, London (1983)
Bodey, G. *Am. J. Medicine* 77 (30/10/84)
Field, D., Adverse Reactions and Side Effects of HIV Treatment, *The J. Naturopathic Med.* 3, 74–6 (1992)
Conge, G. et al. *Reprod. Nutr. Develop.* 20(4A), 929–38 (1980)
Larkin, T. *FDA Consumer* (September 1985)
Chen, G.S. *Am. J. of Acupuncture* 10, 147–53 (1982)
Bjarnason, I. et al. *Lancet* 1171 (24/11/84)
Phillipson, J.D. and Anderson, L.A. *Pharmaceutical J.* 111 (28/7/84)
Mervyn, L. et al. *Biochem. J.* 72, 109 (1959)
Alexander, W.D. *Brit. Med. J.* 2, 501 (1975)
Kaplan, N. *J. American Medical Assoc.* 249, 365–7 (1983)
Editorial, *Brit. Med. J.* 290, 322 (1985)
Dyckner, T. and Wester, P.O. *Practical Cardiology* 10 (15/5/84)
Editorial, *Lancet* 2, 1189–91 (13/12/75)

Chapter 8
Shearer, M.H. *Birth Fam. J.* 6, 119–25 (1974)
Internat. Childbirth Education Assoc., *Special Report*, vol. II (1972)
Gosh, A. and Hudson, F.P. *Lancet* 823 (1977)

Caldeyro-Barcia, R. *Birth Fam. J.* 2, 5–14 (1974)

Macdonald, D. et al. *Am. J. Obst. Gynaecol.* 152, 524–39 (1985)

Brackbill, Y. Obstetric Medication and Infant Development. In Osofsky, (ed.) *Handbook of Infant Development*, Wiley, NY (1971)

Editorial, *Brit. Med. J.* 978–9 (24/4/76)

Marieskind, H.I. *An Evaluation of Caesarian Section in the US*, Office of the Assistant Secretary for Planning and Education/Health, Washington, US Govt. Printing Office (1979)

Harrison, R.F. et al. *Brit. Med. J.* 288, 1971–5 (1980)

Sleep, J. et al. *Brit. Med. J.* 289, 587–90 (1980)

Richards, M.P.M. *Birth Fam. J.* 7, 225–33 (1980)

Collea, J.V. et al. *Am. J. Obstet. Gynaecol.* 131, 186 (1978)

Sosa, R. et al. *New Eng. J. Med.* 303, 597–600 (1980)

Tanzer, D. *The Psychology of Pregnancy and Childbirth: An Investigation of Natural Childbirth*, Ph.D. Thesis, Brandeis University (1967)

Maisels, M.J. et al. *J. American Med. Assoc.* 238, 206 (1977)

Cohen, J. *Birth Fam. J.* 4, 114 (1977)

British Medical J. 287, 81 (1983)

INDEX